Clinical Anaesthesia
Lecture Notes

To Jenny and Sophie, thank you for all the happiness you bring

This title is also available as an e-book.
For more details, please see
www.wiley.com/buy/9781119119821
or scan this QR code:

Clinical Anaesthesia
Lecture Notes

Matthew Gwinnutt

MB ChB (Hons) FRCA
Specialist Trainee in Anaesthesia
Health Education North West
Mersey School of Anaesthesia
UK

Carl Gwinnutt

MB BS MRCS LRCP FRCA
Emeritus Consultant
Salford Royal Hospitals NHS Foundation Trust
Salford, UK

Fifth Edition

WILEY Blackwell

This edition first published 2017 © 2017 by John Wiley & Sons, Ltd.

First edition 1997. © Carl L. Gwinnutt
Second edition 2004. © Carl L. Gwinnutt
Third edition 2008. © Carl L. Gwinnutt
Fourth edition 2012 © 2012 by John Wiley & Sons, Ltd.

Registered Office
John Wiley & Sons, Ltd, The Atrium, Southern Gate, Chichester, West Sussex, PO19 8SQ, UK

Editorial Offices
9600 Garsington Road, Oxford, OX4 2DQ, UK
The Atrium, Southern Gate, Chichester, West Sussex, PO19 8SQ, UK
111 River Street, Hoboken, NJ 07030-5774, USA

For details of our global editorial offices, for customer services and for information about how
to apply for permission to reuse the copyright material in this book please see our website at
www.wiley.com/wiley-blackwell.

Designations used by companies to distinguish their products are often claimed as trademarks. All
brand names and product names used in this book are trade names, service marks, trademarks or
registered trademarks of their respective owners. The publisher is not associated with any product
or vendor mentioned in this book. It is sold on the understanding that the publisher is not engaged
in rendering professional services. If professional advice or other expert assistance is required, the
services of a competent professional should be sought.

The contents of this work are intended to further general scientific research, understanding, and
discussion only and are not intended and should not be relied upon as recommending or promoting
a specific method, diagnosis, or treatment by health science practitioners for any particular patient.
The publisher and the author make no representations or warranties with respect to the accuracy or
completeness of the contents of this work and specifically disclaim all warranties, including without
limitation any implied warranties of fitness for a particular purpose. In view of ongoing research,
equipment modifications, changes in governmental regulations, and the constant flow of information
relating to the use of medicines, equipment, and devices, the reader is urged to review and evaluate the
information provided in the package insert or instructions for each medicine, equipment, or device for,
among other things, any changes in the instructions or indication of usage and for added warnings and
precautions. Readers should consult with a specialist where appropriate. The fact that an organization
or web site is referred to in this work as a citation and/or a potential source of further information does
not mean that the author or the publisher endorses the information the organization or Web site may
provide or recommendations it may make. Further, readers should be aware that internet web sites
listed in this work may have changed or disappeared between when this work was written and when it
is read. No warranty may be created or extended by any promotional statements for this work. Neither
the publisher nor the author shall be liable for any damages arising herefrom.

Library of Congress Cataloging-in-Publication Data

Names: Gwinnutt, Carl L., author. | Gwinnutt, Matthew, author.
Title: Lecture notes. Clinical anaesthesia/Matthew Gwinnutt, Carl Gwinnutt.
Other titles: Clinical anaesthesia
Description: Fifth edition. | Chichester, West Sussex, UK ; Hoboken, NJ :
    John Wiley & Sons Inc., 2017. | Carl Gwinnutt's name appears first on the
    previous edition. | Includes bibliographical references and index.
Identifiers: LCCN 2016011445 | ISBN 9781119119821 (pbk.) | ISBN 9781119119845
    (Adobe PDF) | ISBN 9781119119852 (epub)
Subjects: | MESH: Anesthesia | Anesthetics
Classification: LCC RD81 | NLM WO 200 | DDC 617.9/6-dc23
LC record available at http://lccn.loc.gov/2016011445

A catalogue record for this book is available from the British Library.

Wiley also publishes its books in a variety of electronic formats. Some content that appears in print
may not be available in electronic books.

Cover image: John Wiley and Sons Ltd.

Set in 8.5/11pt Utopia by SPi Global, Pondicherry, India
Printed and bound in Malaysia by Vivar Printing Sdn Bhd

1   2017

Contents

Contributors

Russell Perkins FRCA
Consultant Paediatric Anaesthetist
Royal Manchester Children's Hospital
Manchester, UK

Justin Turner FRCA
Consultant in Anaesthesia and Pain Management
Salford Royal Hospitals NHS Foundation Trust
Salford, UK

Preface

It is only four years since the last edition of this book, but changes continue apace and the time had come to ensure that Lecture Notes, Clinical Anaesthesia reflected these changes and also responded to the feedback received around the previous edition. The first major change is the new Chapter 1, 'An introduction to anaesthesia'. We hope you will take the time to have a look at this, even if only briefly, as we have tried to provide an insight into how the specialty has developed and where it is heading. It is estimated that around 70% of all hospital patients encounter an anaesthetist at some point during their admission, hardly surprising when we consider how broad the scope of the specialty of anaesthesia has become and the numerous professionals working together as part of the team. Therefore, we have approached the task of writing of this edition with the team in mind, and hope that it will be useful not only for medical students but also for trainees in anaesthesia and other acute specialties, trainee physician's assistants in anaesthesia, operating department practitioners and recovery nurses.

As would be expected, the content has been fully updated to reflect areas where there have been changes in clinical practice, new guidelines and new equipment or drugs. We have increased coverage of the perioperative management of the overweight and obese patient to reflect the increasing frequency with which this group of patients is encountered and, in response to numerous requests, we have for the first time included an introduction to some basic aspects of paediatric anaesthesia. Other new topics include an outline of enhanced recovery after surgery (ERAS) and the importance of anaesthetists' non-technical skills (NTS). Given the likely future expansion of anaesthetists into the developing field of perioperative care, we felt it appropriate to keep and expand slightly the chapter detailing the recognition and management of some of the more common perioperative medical emergencies.

Apart from updating the contents, there are two key changes in this edition compared to previous ones. Firstly, to help you take a structured approach to learning about anaesthesia, we have included a series of objectives at the start of each chapter. These are divided into two sections: firstly, the knowledge you should aim to acquire by reading each chapter, and secondly, an indication of the skills that we feel are important and are based upon the former. We hope this will give you a clearer idea of what you should try and achieve during an anaesthetic attachment. For those of you using this book who are not medical students, we feel these learning objectives are equally relevant and achievable.

The second change is an attempt to encourage you to use the vast resources available via the internet. The potential problem with this approach is that there is little quality control over what is available. Therefore, we have only included links to web sites we know, have checked and believe are reliable. For those of you using a hard copy of the book, interesting and useful web sites are numbered within the text, for example [2.2], and the web address is listed in the 'Further information' section at the end of the chapter. For those of you using the e-book, the numbers within the text are hyperlinked directly to an organization's web site or a specific article. We hope you will use this and feel free to feed back your thoughts and comments.

Finally, we close by repeating the same message as in previous editions – we hope that you will enjoy this book but, more importantly, that it helps you provide better care for your patients. If it has, tell your friends, if it hasn't, tell us! We hope that it is improving each time, but it still is and will always remain 'work in progress'.

Acknowledgements

We would like to thank Deltex Medical for Figures 3.16 and 3.17. Figure 3.7 is from McGuire and Younger, 2010 (see Further information in Chapter 3), with permission of Oxford University Press on behalf of the *British Journal of Anaesthesia*.

Figure 5.12 is reproduced with permission of Dr P. Ross and I am grateful to Dr J. Corcoran for his help and advice with transversus abdominis plane blocks and Figure 6.1.

Figures 9.8, 9.9, 9.10 and 9.11 are reproduced with kind permission from the Resuscitation Council (UK) and Dr Michael Scott.

Thanks are due to the Difficult Airway Society for Figure 5.9, the National Tracheostomy Safety Project for Figures 9.3 and 9.4, and to Dr David Pitcher for his guidance on 'Decisions about cardiopulmonary resuscitation'.

We would also like to express our gratitude to Dr Richard Morgan, Professor Gary Smith and Dr Jas Soar for their contributions to the previous editions, some of which by necessity have been included in this edition.

Abbreviations

AAGBI	Association of Anaesthetists of Great Britain and Ireland	CSF	cerebrospinal fluid
ABG	arterial blood gas	CT	computed tomography
ABW	adjusted body weight	CTPA	computed tomography pulmonary angiography
ACD-A	anticoagulant citrate dextrose solution A	CVC	central venous catheter
ACE-I	angiotensin converting enzyme inhibitor	CVP	central venous pressure
ACS	acute coronary syndrome	CVS	cardiovascular system
ADH	antidiuretic hormone	CXR	chest X-ray
AIM	Acute Illness Management	DAS	Difficult Airway Society
AKI	acute kidney injury	DBP	diastolic blood pressure
ALERT	Acute Life-threatening Event Recognition and Treatment	DBS	double-burst simulation
		DNACPR	do not attempt cardiopulmonary resuscitation
ALS	Advanced Life Support	DS	degrees of substitution
AMI	acute myocardial infarction	DVT	deep venous thrombosis
ANTT	antiseptic no-touch technique	ECF	extracellular fluid
APL	adjustable pressure limiting	ECG	electrocardiogram
APLS	Advanced Paediatric Life Support	EEG	electroencephalograph
ARDS	acute respiratory distress syndrome	EMLA	eutectic mixture of local anaesthetics
ASA	American Society of Anesthesiologists	ENT	ear, nose and throat
AT	anaerobic threshold	EPLS	European Paediatric Life Support
ATN	acute tubular necrosis	ETC	European Trauma Course
AV	atrioventricular	ETT	exercise tolerance test
BIS	bispectral index	EWS	Early Warning Score
BMI	body mass index	FAST	focused assessment with sonography in trauma
BNF	*British National Formulary*		
BiPAP	bilevel positive airway pressure	FBC	full blood count
BP	blood pressure	FEEL	focused echocardiography in emergency life support
BTS	British Thoracic Society		
CAP	community-acquired pneumonia	FEV_1	forced expiratory volume in 1 second
CCrISP	Care of the Critically Ill Surgical Patient	FFP	fresh frozen plasma
CCU	coronary care unit	FICM	Faculty of Intensive Care Medicine
CEPOD	Confidential Enquiry into Perioperative Death	FiO_2	fractional inspired oxygen concentration
CNS	central nervous system	FRC	functional residual capacity
CO_2	carbon dioxide	FRCA	Fellow of the Royal College of Anaesthetists
COPD	chronic obstructive pulmonary disease		
COX	cyclo-oxygenase	FVC	forced vital capacity
CPAP	continuous positive airway pressure	GCS	Glasgow Coma Scale
CPR	cardiopulmonary resuscitation	GFR	glomerular filtration rate
CPX	cardiopulmonary exercise	GI	gastrointestinal
CRP	C-reactive protein	GTN	glyceryl trinitrate
CRT	capillary refill time	HAFOE	high-airflow oxygen enrichment

HAP	hospital-acquired pneumonia
Hb	haemoglobin
HbA1c	glycosylated haemoglobin
HDU	high-dependency unit
HIV	human immunodeficiency virus
HR	heart rate
HRT	hormone replacement therapy
5-HT	5-hydroxytryptamine
HTLV	human T-cell lymphotrophic virus
IBW	ideal body weight
ICF	intracellular fluid
ICM	intensive care medicine
ICP	intracranial pressure
ICU	intensive care unit
I:E ratio	inspiratory:expiratory ratio
ILMA	intubating LMA
IM	intramuscular
INR	international normalized ratio
IPPV	intermittent positive pressure ventilation
IR	immediate release
ITU	intensive therapy unit
IV	intravenous
IVC	inferior vena cava
IVRA	intravenous regional anaesthesia
JVP	jugular venous pressure
K^+	potassium ions
kPa	kilopascals
LA	local anaesthetic
LBBB	left bundle branch block
LBW	lean body weight
LED	light-emitting diode
LFT	liver function test
LMA	laryngeal mask airway
LMWH	low molecular weight heparin
LP	lumbar puncture
LSD	lysergic acid diethylamide
LVF	left ventricular failure
MAC	minimum alveolar concentration
MAP	mean arterial pressure
MET	metabolic equivalent; medical emergency team
MH	malignant hyperpyrexia
MHRA	Medicines and Healthcare products Regulatory Agency
MI	myocardial infarction
MODS	multiple organ dysfunction syndrome
MR	modified release

MRI	magnetic resonance imaging
Na^+	sodium ions
NCEPOD	National Confidential Enquiry into Patient Outcome and Death
NEWS	National Early Warning Score
NIBP	non-invasive blood pressure
NICE	National Institute for Health and Care Excellence
NMDA	N-methyl-D-aspartate
N_2O	nitrous oxide
NPSA	National Patient Safety Agency
NSAID	non-steroidal anti-inflammatory drug
NSTEMI	non-ST segment elevation myocardial infarction
NYHA	New York Heart Association
OCP	oral contraceptive pill
ODP	operating department practitioner
OHS	obesity hypoventilation syndrome
OLV	one-lung ventilation
OSA	obstructive sleep apnoea
OSAHS	obstructive sleep apnoea and hypopnoea syndrome
OS-MRS	Obesity Surgery Mortality Risk Score
OTC	over the counter
PA(A)	physician's assistant (anaesthesia)
$PaCO_2$	arterial partial pressure of carbon dioxide
PACU	postanaesthesia care unit
PCA	patient-controlled anaesthesia
PCI	percutaneous coronary intervention
PCV	pressure-controlled ventilation
PDPH	postdural puncture headache
PE	pulmonary embolism
PEA	pulseless electrical activity
PEEP	positive end expiratory pressure
PEF	peak expiratory flow
PEFR	peak expiratory flow rate
PMGV	piped medical gas and vacuum system
PaO_2	arterial partial pressure of oxygen
POCT	point of care testing
PONV	postoperative nausea and vomiting
PPCI	primary percutaneous coronary intervention
PPI	proton pump inhibitor
psi	pounds per square inch
PSV	pressure support ventilation
PT	prothrombin time
pVT	pulseless ventricular tachycardia
RBBB	right bundle branch block

ROSC	return of spontaneous circulation	TBW	total body weight
RRT	renal replacement therapy	TCI	target-controlled infusion
RSI	rapid-sequence induction	TIVA	total intravenous anaesthesia
RSVP	Reason, Story, Vital signs, Plan	TOF	train-of-four
SBAR	Situation, Background, Assessment, Response	TTE	transthoracic echocardiography
SBP	systolic blood pressure	U&E	urea and electrolytes
SGA	supraglottic airway	VCO_2	carbon dioxide production
SIRS	systemic inflammatory response syndrome	VF	ventricular fibrillation
SOBA	Society for Obesity and Bariatric Anaesthesia	VIE	vacuum-insulated evaporator
SpO_2	peripheral oxygen saturation	VO_2	oxygen consumption
STEMI	ST segment elevation myocardial infarction	V/Q	ventilation/perfusion ratio
SVC	superior vena cava	VT	ventricular tachycardia
TAP	transversus abdominis plane	VTE	venous thromboembolism
		WBC	white blood cell
		WHO	World Health Organization

About the companion website

Don't forget to visit the companion website for this book:

www.lecturenoteseries.com/anaesthesia

There you will find valuable material designed to enhance your learning, including:

- Interactive true/false questions
- Interactive short-answer questions
- A list of further reading and resources.

Scan this QR code to visit the companion website:

An introduction to anaesthesia

General anaesthesia

Nitrous oxide was first synthesized by Joseph Priestley in 1772, and had been known to have analgesic properties since the turn of the nineteenth century, but it was mostly used as a recreational drug (laughing gas). Horace Wells, a dentist in Connecticut, USA, noticed that an assistant under the influence of the gas suffered a significant injury to his shin, but appeared unaware until later. Wells subsequently had one of his wisdom teeth extracted painlessly whilst inhaling nitrous oxide and went on to use the gas in his own practice in 1844. Unfortunately, in 1845, when invited to demonstrate the effects on a patient having a dental extraction at Harvard Medical School, the patient complained of pain and Wells was denounced as a fraud. These early administrations of nitrous oxide carried the risk of severe hypoxia as it was given in close to 100% concentration to obtain an adequate effect. This was solved in the late 1860s, when it was supplied in cylinders under pressure and given in conjunction with 20% oxygen, which lead to an increase in its use.

The first successful public demonstration of painless surgery occurred on 16 October 1846 at Massachusetts General Hospital. William Thomas Green Morton, a dentist, presided over the inhalation of ether vapour (diethyl ether, $(C_2H_5)_2O$) by Edward Abbott while John Warren, the senior surgeon, removed a tumour from Abbott's jaw. It wasn't until a few weeks later that a name for the state induced was proposed by Oliver Wendell Holmes, Professor of Anatomy and Physiology at Harvard University: 'anaesthesia', from the Greek *an* (without) and *aisthesis*

(sensation). Compare the simple device used by Morton (Figure 1.1a) with one of today's anaesthesia machines (Figure 1.1b).

Unsurprisingly, news of this discovery spread rapidly and on 19 December 1846, Dr Francis Boott, a physician in London, encouraged James Robinson, a dentist, to give ether to a patient for the extraction of a wisdom tooth. The result was so impressive that Dr Boott persuaded Robert Liston, Professor of Surgery at the University of London, to allow ether to be given during the amputation of Frederick Churchill's leg, which proved to be a complete success.

Despite the spreading popularity of ether anaesthesia, it was acknowledged that there were problems controlling the dose as the liquid cooled as it vaporized. The first person to apply scientific methodology to giving ether vapour was John Snow, a London physician who invented several pieces of equipment to allow the delivery of known concentrations. He subsequently used chloroform in preference to ether, and in April 1853 successfully gave chloroform to Queen Victoria during the birth of her eighth child, Leopold. He repeated this process in April 1857 at the birth of Victoria's last child, Beatrice. By the end of the nineteenth century, combinations of nitrous oxide, ether and chloroform, with oxygen, were being used widely to achieve anaesthesia.

Over the next 50 years a number of other inhaled anaesthetics were introduced, including ethyl chloride, cyclopropane and trichloroethylene but ether, chloroform and nitrous oxide dominated. The next major breakthrough came when in 1951 Charles Suckling, working at Imperial Chemical Industries (ICI) in Manchester, synthesized halothane and in 1956 it was first used clinically by Michael Johnstone at the Manchester Royal Infirmary. This was the start of the modern era of inhaled anaesthetics and the next 40 years saw the synthesis of several complex halogenated ethers, which yielded the drugs in use today: isoflurane, sevoflurane and desflurane.

Clinical Anaesthesia: Lecture Notes, Fifth Edition. Matthew Gwinnutt and Carl Gwinnutt.
© 2017 John Wiley & Sons, Ltd. Published 2017 by John Wiley & Sons, Ltd.
Companion website: www.lecturenoteseries.com/anaesthesia

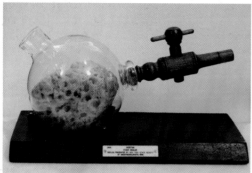

(a)

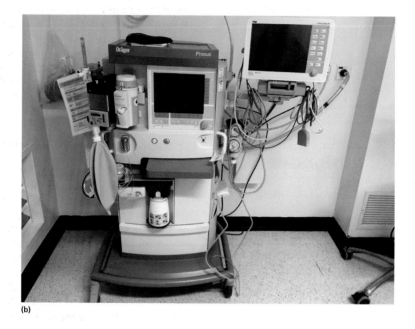

(b)

Figure 1.1 (a) Replica of the ether inhaler used by William Morton to give the first public demonstration of general anaesthesia, 16 October 1846, in Massachusetts General Hospital. Reproduced with kind permission of the Association of anaesthetists of Great Britain and Northern Ireland. (b) Modern integrated anaesthesia system.

The other key discovery that revolutionized general anaesthesia was of neuromuscular blocking drugs or 'muscle relaxants'. Amazonian Indians were known to apply a plant extract called curare to the tips of their arrowheads that left their prey paralysed. In 1812, it was shown that artificial ventilation could keep animals alive until the poison wore off and they made a full recovery. The science behind this observation was revealed in 1850 by the French physiologist Claude Bernard when he showed that curare acted at the neuromuscular junction. In 1900, the anti-curare effects of physostigmine were described and so the effects of curare could be reversed when needed,

rather than waiting for spontaneous recovery. Interestingly, the first clinical use of curare was not in anaesthesia, but in the treatment of tetanus in 1934. It was not until 1942 that Harold Griffith and Enid Johnson at Magill University, Montreal, used curare as part of their anaesthetic for a patient undergoing an appendicectomy. Curare (d-tubocurarine) was first introduced into clinical practice in England by Gray and Halton in Liverpool in 1946. Five years later suxamethonium (succinylcholine) was introduced into clinical practice, again after a considerable delay since its first description in 1906. In 1966, pancuronium, the first synthetic muscle relaxant, was introduced, followed in the early 1980s by vecuronium and atracurium.

Finally, no writing on the history of general anaesthesia is complete without a brief mention of tracheal intubation. This evolved from the use of metal tubes in the eighteenth century which were passed into the trachea to aid with resuscitation. It was William MacEwen, a Glasgow surgeon, who deliberately first introduced a flexible metallic tube into a patient's trachea through which chloroform in air was given. The patient required the removal of a tumour at the base of their tongue and would otherwise have needed a tracheostomy. Numerous similar techniques followed, but it was Magill and Rowbotham who first passed tubes into the trachea to secure the airway and allow unhindered access to the face and airway to perform reconstructive surgery. The endotracheal tubes that Magill went on to develop were reusable, made from rubber, and became the universal standard for over 40 years. They have now been replaced by single-use tubes made from polyvinyl chloride (PVC).

Local and regional anaesthesia

The Indians in Bolivia and Peru had chewed the leaves of the bush *Erythroxylum coca* for its stimulant properties which enabled them to go on prolonged hunting trips without tiring. In the mid-1850s, the active ingredient, an alkaloid named cocaine, had been extracted and was investigated by Freud as a remedy for morphine addiction and use in psychoneurotic patients. Aware of the effects of cocaine in 'deadening' mucous membranes, he asked a colleague, Carl Koller, an eye surgeon in Vienna, to carry out some investigations. Koller experimented firstly on animals, then himself and friends and finally on patients. He showed that instilling cocaine into the conjunctival sac made eye operations completely painless for the first time. By the 1890s, cocaine was being used for nerve and plexus blocks, but many of the pioneers were unaware of its addictive properties and experimented upon themselves, becoming addicts in the process. This problem lead to the development of safer alternatives and by the turn of the twentieth century, stovaine and procaine (novocaine) were widely used. Lignocaine (lidocaine) was synthesized in 1943 and first used clinically in 1948 and bupivacaine appeared in 1963.

The development of central neural blockade or spinal anaesthesia came about by accident in 1885.

James Corning, a New York neurologist, accidentally injected cocaine intrathecally in a dog and, noting its profound effect, repeated the injection in a patient. He coined the term 'spinal anaesthesia', suggesting it might have a use for surgery. In 1898, August Bier, a German surgeon, gave the first deliberate spinal anaesthetic for surgery with cocaine. Having repeated the technique successfully on a further small group of patients, Bier allowed his assistant to give intrathecal cocaine to him, thereby proving his faith in the technique. The introduction of stovaine and procaine eliminated the risk of toxicity and addiction, and the popularity of spinal anaesthesia spread.

Epidural anaesthesia soon followed, firstly using a technique of giving the drugs via the caudal route. The lumbar route, which is widely used today, was popularized in Europe in the 1930s by the Italian surgeon Achille Dogliotti and in the UK in the 1940s by Charles Massey Dawkins. Shortly after, the first use of a catheter in the epidural space to allow continual analgesia was described.

Anaesthesia today

Anaesthesia has progressed from the early days of dripping ether or chloroform onto a piece of gauze held over the patient's face. Lack of control and the use of relatively toxic drugs meant that effects were often unpredictable and complications, including death, were not uncommon. Monitoring the patient meant feeling their pulse, looking at their colour and observing rate and depth of breathing. Training was done 'on the job' and there were no standards or regulations.

Currently in the United Kingdom, doctors who have completed their medical training then undergo a further seven years training to become anaesthetists. During this time, they take part in a structured training programme and sit postgraduate examinations to become a Fellow of the Royal College of Anaesthetists (FRCA) [1.1]. In addition, many also undertake additional subspecialization training, for example in critical care, pain management, cardiothoracic, neurosurgical or paediatric anaesthesia. Anaesthetists form the largest group of specialists within the NHS and it is estimated that over 60% of patients will encounter an anaesthetist during their time in hospital.

Today, anaesthetists must have a detailed understanding of physiology, pharmacology, anatomy and physics. This knowledge is essential; during a routine anaesthetic (if such a thing exists!) a wide variety of anaesthetic techniques, sophisticated equipment and drugs is available and the correct combination of these must be used to achieve the effect required. Many of the drugs used and the 'stress' of surgery have significant effects on the patient's physiology. As a result, patients must be closely monitored; during most operations the anaesthetist will use a wide variety of different electronic monitors which give information on the physiological changes taking place, concentrations of anaesthetic drugs and oxygen and performance of ventilators. Such advances have made modern anaesthesia extremely safe; since the 1960s, mortality attributable to anaesthesia has fallen 10-fold, from 357 to 34 per million anaesthetics.

Today's anaesthetist no longer works in isolation giving patients anaesthesia to allow surgery; they work as part of a team and take on a greater number of roles and responsibilities than ever before.

The preoperative assessment

Although not all patients need to be seen by an anaesthetist in a preoperative assessment clinic, all patients do need to be assessed by an appropriately trained individual. This role is frequently undertaken by nurses. They will take a history, examine the patient and order investigations, according to the local protocol. The primary aim is to identify those patients at low risk of complications during anaesthesia and surgery and who can be listed safely without the need to be assessed at this point by an anaesthetist. Clearly, not all patients achieve this goal and will need further investigations prior to being seen by an anaesthetist in the clinic.

The anaesthetic assistant

Many surgical procedures performed today would not be possible without the advances that have been made in anaesthetic drugs, techniques and equipment available to anaesthetists. However, it is important to recognize the fact that, unlike even 50 years ago, anaesthetists are now the leaders of a team of healthcare professionals caring for patients pre-, intra- and postoperatively. Whilst working in the operating theatre, they are always assisted by either an operating department practitioner (ODP) or an anaesthetic nurse. These individuals have undergone a training programme in order to assist the anaesthetist in the safe delivery of anaesthesia, and have a wide variety of responsibilities, from checking and preparing equipment to assisting in the resuscitation of patients.

Physicians' assistant (anaesthesia)

The latest member of the anaesthesia team, introduced in 2004, is the physicians' assistant (anaesthesia) (PA(A)). PA(A)s are fully trained professionals who have completed a postgraduate diploma and work under the direction and supervision of a consultant anaesthetist, a typical situation being where one consultant anaesthetist supervises two PA(A)s or one PA(A) and an anaesthetic trainee. The roles of the PA(A)s are generally to help increase operating theatre efficiency by allowing quicker turnround between operations, thereby increasing the throughput of patients. They have also found roles in the preoperative assessment clinic, cardiopulmonary exercise testing and cardiac arrest team.

Immediate postoperative care

Any patient who has received an anaesthetic will spend some time in a postoperative or postanaesthesia care unit (PACU), often simply known as the 'recovery unit'. This is a specialized area where patients are closely monitored by specially trained nurses or ODPs for a period of time immediately after anaesthesia and surgery. The PACU was developed in response to the significant number of preventable deaths that occurred during recovery from anaesthesia and surgery. Nowadays, any patient who is not returned immediately to a critical care area will spend time in a PACU where their vital signs will be monitored and drugs given for analgesia and relief of nausea and vomiting. Ultimately, the anaesthetist retains overall responsibility for this aspect of patient care until discharged to a ward.

Anaesthetists in critical care

In 1952, Copenhagen suffered a devastating polio epidemic that resulted in hundreds of patients experiencing respiratory and bulbar failure. Many only survived because around 1000 medical and dental students were recruited to ventilate manually these patients, often for several weeks, via tracheostomies (Figure 1.2). As a result, the following year, Bjorn Ibsen, the anaesthetist who had suggested this solution for the management of these patients, set up the first intensive care unit (ICU) in Europe and many consider him to be the 'father' of intensive care.

During the 1960s and 1970s, ICUs were gradually established in the United Kingdom and Professor

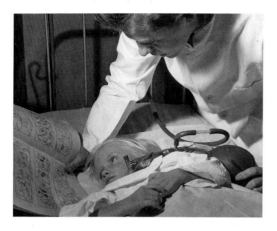

Figure 1.2 Young child being ventilated by hand via a tracheostomy during the 1952 polio epidemic in Copenhagen. Reproduced with kind permission of the Medical Museum, University of Copenhagen.

Ron Bradley, who was probably the first full-time intensive care clinician, ran the ICU at St Thomas' Hospital in London. As hospitals established intensive care units, many were run by anaesthetists by virtue of their training and experience of caring for ventilated patients. Today, intensive care has become a multidisciplinary specialty with dedicated ICU nurses, physiotherapists, pharmacists, dieticians, technicians, radiologists and microbiologists. The dedicated staff and specialized equipment in the modern ICU allow support or even temporary replacement of the function of many of a patient's organ systems in the face of critical illness and injury. It is this knowledge and skill that underpins intensive care medicine (ICM). In the UK, intensive care has now become a stand-alone specialty, with the formation of the Faculty of Intensive Care Medicine (FICM) in 2010, with a separate training programme as of 2012. As a result, training in ICM is now accessible to staff from other medical specialties, for example respiratory medicine, renal medicine, cardiology and emergency medicine, as well as from the more traditional route via anaesthesia [1.2] [1.3].

Anaesthetists in pain management

The purpose of anaesthesia is to enable pain-free surgery. This has led to anaesthetists using their skills to become involved in the management of pain in both the acute and chronic setting. In 1990, a joint publication from the Royal College of Surgeons of England and the College of Anaesthetists (as it was then), *Pain after Surgery*, highlighted the need for hospitals to develop services to ensure adequate pain relief, and reduce the incidence of side-effects and the associated postoperative morbidity and mortality. Anaesthetists have taken a leading role in the multidisciplinary acute pain teams that are now established in hospitals to achieve this.

Chronic pain management in both cancer and non-malignant conditions is also an area where anaesthetists have developed a subspecialty interest. Chronic pain affects all ages and all parts of a patients' wellbeing and successful management requires a biopsychosocial assessment of all the aspects of life affected by pain.

To achieve this, anaesthetists were at the forefront of the establishment of 'pain clinics', now more appropriately called pain medicine or pain management. These allow patients to be treated on an outpatient basis where, in addition to assessment and psychological support, injections, neuromodulation and participation in rehabilitation teams are used to provide individual pain management programmes.

The Faculty of Pain Medicine of the Royal College of Anaesthetists was established in 2007 to provide guidance on standards in pain medicine. The Faculty also sets the training requirements and an examination for those new to the specialty and intending to pursue a career with an interest in pain management.

Anaesthesia in the future

Although the safety of surgery and anaesthesia has improved dramatically over the past 50 years, evidence suggests that patients suffer a significant amount of avoidable harm after major surgery. However, much of this harm is preventable by intervention before or after surgery, for example preoperative correction of anaemia, postoperative analgesia and fluid balance. Traditionally, the surgical team has had responsibility for the care of patients in this period. Increasingly, surgeons are focusing on training in the technical aspects of more complex procedures, and patients have complex medical needs. It is falling to other specialists to provide care for patients in the perioperative period. As a result, the subspecialty of perioperative medicine is beginning to evolve and it is anaesthetists who are taking the lead thanks to their unique combination of training and experience.

The anaesthetist of the future is likely to play an increasing role through the patient's journey, from the point of decision to operate until discharge home, to ensure the individual needs of each patient are met and the potential for harm minimized.

FURTHER INFORMATION

[1.1] www.rcoa.ac.uk
[1.2] www.ficm.ac.uk
[1.3] www.ics.ac.uk

2

Anaesthetic assessment and preparation for surgery

Learning objectives

After reading this chapter you should understand the principles of:

☐ The role of the preoperative assessment clinic

☐ Comorbidities that may impact on the conduct or risk of anaesthesia

☐ Which investigations are necessary prior to anaesthesia

☐ Airway assessment and indicators of potential difficulties with tracheal intubation

☐ Risks associated with anaesthesia

☐ Obtaining consent for both general and regional anaesthesia

Apply this knowledge when practising the following skills:

☐ Taking a history, paying particular attention to those features that may impact on the conduct of anaesthesia

☐ Examining a patient, paying particular attention to assessment of their airway

☐ Constructing an anaesthetic plan in conjunction with an anaesthetist

The nature of anaesthetists' training and experience makes them uniquely qualified to assess the inherent risks of anaesthetizing each individual patient. Ideally, every patient should be seen by an anaesthetist prior to surgery to identify, manage and minimize these risks. Traditionally, this occurred when the patient was admitted, usually the day before an elective surgical procedure. However, if at this time the patient was found to have any significant comorbidity, surgery was often postponed but with insufficient time to admit a different patient, leading to wasted operating time. Increasingly, in attempts to improve efficiency, patients are admitted on the day of their planned surgical procedure. This further reduces the opportunity for an adequate anaesthetic assessment, limits the investigations that can be done and virtually prevents optimization of any comorbidities. This has led to significant changes in the preoperative management of patients undergoing elective surgery, including the introduction of clinics specifically for anaesthetic assessment. A variety of

Clinical Anaesthesia: Lecture Notes, Fifth Edition. Matthew Gwinnutt and Carl Gwinnutt.
© 2017 John Wiley & Sons, Ltd. Published 2017 by John Wiley & Sons, Ltd.
Companion website: www.lecturenoteseries.com/anaesthesia

models of 'preoperative' or 'anaesthetic assessment' clinic exist; the following is intended to outline their principal functions. Those who require greater detail are advised to consult the document produced by the Association of Anaesthetists of Great Britain and Ireland (AAGBI) [2.1].

The preoperative assessment clinic

Stage 1

Although not all patients need to be seen by an anaesthetist in a preoperative assessment clinic, all patients do need to be assessed by an appropriately trained individual. This role is frequently undertaken by nurses who may take a history, examine the patient, and order investigations (see later) according to the local protocol. The primary aim is to identify those patients at low risk of complications during anaesthesia and surgery. This includes patients who:

- have no coexisting medical problems;
- have a coexisting medical problem that is well controlled and does not impair daily activities, such as hypertension;
- do not require any or require only baseline investigations (Table 2.1);
- have no history of, or predicted, anaesthetic difficulties;
- require surgery for which complications are minimal.

Having fulfilled these criteria, patients can then be listed for surgery. At this stage, the patient will usually be given preliminary information about anaesthesia, often in the form of an explanatory leaflet. On admission, patients will be seen by a member of the surgical team to ensure that there have not been any significant changes since attending the clinic, reaffirm consent and mark the surgical site if appropriate. The anaesthetist will:

- confirm the findings at the preoperative assessment;
- check the results of any baseline investigations;
- explain the options for anaesthesia appropriate for the procedure;
- obtain consent for anaesthesia;
- have the ultimate responsibility for deciding whether it is safe to proceed.

Stage 2

Clearly, not all patients are as described above. Common reasons for this are:

- coexisting medical problems that impair activities of daily living;
- the discovery of previously undiagnosed medical problems, such as diabetes or hypertension;
- medical conditions that are less than optimally managed, such as angina, chronic obstructive pulmonary disease (COPD);
- abnormal baseline investigations.

These patients will need to be sent for further investigations – for example, an electrocardiogram (ECG),

Table 2.1 Baseline investigations in patients with no evidence of concurrent disease (ASA I).

Age of patient	Minor surgery	Intermediate surgery	Major surgery	Major 'plus' surgery
16–39	Nil	Nil	FBC	FBC, RFT
Consider	Nil	Nil	RFT, BS	Clotting, BS
40–59	Nil	Nil	FBC	FBC, RFT
Consider	ECG	ECG, FBC, BS	ECG, BS, RFT	ECG, BS, clotting
60–79	Nil	FBC	FBC, ECG, RFT	FBC, RFT, ECG
Consider	ECG	ECG, BS, RFT	BS, CXR	BS, clotting, CXR
≥80	ECG	FBC, ECG	FBC, ECG, RFT	FBC, RFT, ECG
Consider	FBC, RFT	RFT, BS	BS, CXR, clotting	BS, clotting, CXR

BS, random blood glucose; CXR, chest X-ray; ECG, electrocardiogram; FBC, full blood count; RFT, renal function tests, to include sodium, potassium, urea and creatinine.
Clotting to include prothrombin time (PT), activated partial thromboplastin time (APTT), international normalized ratio (INR).
Source: Courtesy of National Institute for Health and Clinical Excellence.

pulmonary function tests, echocardiography – or will be referred to the appropriate specialist for advice or management before being reassessed. The findings of further investigations dictate whether or not the patient needs to be seen by an anaesthetist.

Stage 3

Patients who will need to be seen by an anaesthetist in the preoperative clinic are those who:

- have concurrent disease that impairs activities of daily living (ASA 3, see later);
- are known to have had previous anaesthetic difficulties, such as difficult intubation, allergies to drugs;
- are predicted to have the potential for difficulties, for example morbid obesity or a family history of prolonged apnoea after anaesthesia;
- are to undergo complex surgery with or without planned admission to the intensive care unit (ICU) postoperatively.

The consultation will allow the anaesthetist to:

- make a full assessment of the patient's medical condition;
- evaluate the results of any investigations or advice from other specialists;
- request any additional investigations;
- review any previous anaesthetics given;
- decide on the most appropriate anaesthetic technique, for example general or regional anaesthesia;
- begin the consent process, explaining and documenting:
  o the anaesthetic options available and the potential side-effects;
  o the risks associated with anaesthesia;
- discuss plans for postoperative care.

These patients will also be seen by their anaesthetist on admission, who will confirm that there have not been any significant changes since they were seen in the clinic, answer any further questions that the patient may have about anaesthesia, and obtain informed consent.

The ultimate aim of this process is to ensure that once patients are admitted for surgery, their intended procedures are not cancelled as a result of them being deemed 'unfit' or because their medical conditions have not been adequately investigated. Clearly, the time between the patient being seen in the assessment clinic and the date of admission for surgery cannot be excessive; 4–6 weeks is usually acceptable.

The anaesthetic assessment

The anaesthetic assessment consists of taking a history from, and examining, each patient, followed by any appropriate investigations. When performed by non-anaesthetic staff, a protocol is often used to ensure all the relevant areas are covered. This section concentrates on features of particular relevance to the anaesthetist.

Present and past medical history

For the anaesthetist, the patient's medical history relating to the cardiovascular and respiratory systems are relatively more important.

Cardiovascular system

Enquire specifically about symptoms of:

- ischaemic heart disease;
- heart failure;
- hypertension;
- valvular heart disease;
- conduction defects, arrhythmias;
- peripheral vascular disease, previous deep venous thrombosis (DVT) or pulmonary embolus (PE).

Patients with a proven history of myocardial infarction (MI) are at a greater risk of further infarction perioperatively. The risk of reinfarction falls as the time elapsed since the original event increases. The time when the risk falls to an acceptable level, or to that of a patient with no previous history of MI, varies between patients. For a patient with an uncomplicated MI and a normal exercise tolerance test (ETT), elective surgery may only need to be delayed by 6–8 weeks. Patients should be asked about frequency, severity and predictability of angina attacks. Frequently occurring or unpredictable attacks suggest unstable angina. This should prompt further investigation and optimization of antianginal therapy prior to proceeding with anaesthesia. The American Heart Association has produced guidance for perioperative cardiovascular evaluation (see Further information section).

Heart failure is one of the most important predictors of perioperative complications, mainly as an increased risk of perioperative cardiac morbidity and mortality. Its severity is best described using a recognized scale, such as the New York Heart Association (NYHA) classification (Table 2.2).

Table 2.2 New York Heart Association (NYHA) classification of cardiac function compared to the Specific Activity Scale.

NYHA functional classification		Specific Activity Scale classification
Class I	Cardiac disease without limitation of physical activity	Can perform activities requiring ≥7 METs. Jog/walk at 5 mph, ski, play squash or basketball, shovel soil
	No fatigue, palpitations, dyspnoea or angina	
Class II	Cardiac disease resulting in slight limitation of physical activity	Can perform activities requiring ≥5 but <7 METs
	Asymptomatic at rest, ordinary physical activity causes fatigue, palpitations, dyspnoea or angina	Walk at 4 mph on level ground, garden, rake, weed, have sexual intercourse without stopping
Class III	Cardiac disease causing marked limitation of physical activity	Can perform activities requiring ≥2 but <5 METs
	Asymptomatic at rest, less than ordinary activity causes fatigue, palpitations, dyspnoea or angina	Perform most household chores, play golf, push the lawnmower, shower
Class IV	Cardiac disease limiting any physical activity. Symptoms of heart failure or angina at rest, increased with any physical activity	Patients cannot perform activities requiring ≥2 METs. Cannot dress without stopping because of symptoms; cannot perform any class III activities

MET, metabolic equivalent.

Untreated or poorly controlled hypertension may lead to exaggerated cardiovascular responses during anaesthesia. Both hypertension and hypotension can be precipitated, which increase the risk of myocardial and cerebral ischaemia. The severity of hypertension will determine the action required. Where possible, blood pressure results obtained in the clinic should be confirmed with home blood pressure monitoring.

- *Stage 1 hypertension:* clinic blood pressure is 140/90 mmHg or higher. No evidence that delaying surgery for treatment affects outcome.
- *Stage 2 hypertension:* clinic blood pressure is 160/90 mmHg or higher. Consider review of treatment. If unchanged, requires close monitoring to avoid swings during anaesthesia and surgery.
- *Stage 3 hypertension:* clinic systolic blood pressure 180 mmHg or higher, diastolic 110 mmHg or higher. With a blood pressure this high, elective surgery should be postponed and the patient referred for treatment, due to the significant risk of myocardial ischaemia, arrhythmias and intracerebral haemorrhage. If surgery is urgent (e.g. cancer) or emergency, the blood pressure will require acute control in conjunction with invasive monitoring. If the patient is known to suffer from hypertension, a check with their

general practitioner should be made to find out their normal blood pressure (BP) outside of the hospital environment.

Respiratory system

Enquire specifically about symptoms of:

- COPD;
- asthma;
- infection;
- restrictive lung disease.

Patients with preexisting lung disease are at increased risk of postoperative chest infections, particularly if they are also obese or undergoing upper abdominal or thoracic surgery. If an acute upper respiratory tract infection is present, anaesthesia and surgery should be postponed unless it is for a life-threatening condition.

Assessment of exercise tolerance

Exercise capacity has long been recognized as a good predictor of postoperative morbidity and mortality. This is because surgery provokes similar physiological responses to exercising, namely an increase in tissue oxygen demand necessitating an increase in cardiac output and oxygen delivery. An indication of cardiac and respiratory reserves can be obtained by asking the patient about their ability to perform everyday physical activities before having to stop because of symptoms of chest pain, shortness of breath, etc. For example:

- Could you run for a bus?
- How far can you walk uphill?
- How far can you walk on the flat?
- Are you able to do the shopping?
- How many stairs can you climb before stopping?
- Are you able to do housework?
- Are you able to care for yourself?

The problem with such questions is that they are very subjective, dependent on the patient's motivation, and patients often tend to overestimate their abilities!

The assessment can be made more objective by reference to the Specific Activity Scale (see Table 2.2). Common physical activities are graded in terms of their metabolic equivalents of activity or METs, with 1 MET being the energy (or, more accurately, oxygen) used at rest. The more strenuous the activity, the greater the number of METs used. This is not specific for each patient but serves as a useful guide, and once again relies on the patient's assessment of their activity.

Other important considerations

- *Indigestion, heartburn and reflux:* possibility of a hiatus hernia. If exacerbated on bending forward or lying flat, this increases the risk of regurgitation and aspiration.
- *Rheumatoid disease:* limited movement of joints makes positioning for surgery difficult. Cervical spine and temporomandibular joint involvement may complicate airway management. There is often a chronic anaemia.
- *Diabetes:* an increased incidence of ischaemic heart disease, renal dysfunction and autonomic and peripheral neuropathy. There is also an increased risk of perioperative complications, particularly disruption of glycaemic control, hypotension and infections.
- *Neuromuscular disorders:* poor respiratory function (forced vital capacity (FVC) <1 L) predisposes to chest infection and increases the chance of needing ventilatory support postoperatively. Poor bulbar function predisposes to

aspiration. Care is needed when using muscle relaxants. Consider regional anaesthesia.
- *Chronic renal failure:* anaemia and electrolyte abnormalities. Altered drug excretion restricts the choice of anaesthetic drugs. Surgery and dialysis treatments need to be coordinated.
- *Jaundice (associated with liver dysfunction):* coagulopathy. Altered drug metabolism and excretion. Care is needed especially with use of opioids.

Previous anaesthetics and operations

These have usually occurred in hospitals or occasionally, in the past, dental surgeries. Enquire about any perioperative problems, such as nausea, vomiting, dreams, awareness, jaundice. Ask if any information was given postoperatively, for example difficulty with intubation or delayed recovery. Whenever possible, check the records of previous anaesthetics to rule out or clarify problems such as difficulties with intubation, allergy to drugs given or adverse reactions (such as malignant hyperpyrexia, see later). Some patients may have been issued with a 'Medic-Alert' type bracelet or similar device giving details or a contact number. Details of previous surgical procedures may reveal potential anaesthetic problems, for example cardiac, pulmonary or cervical spine surgery.

Family history

All patients should be asked whether any family members have experienced problems with anaesthesia; for example, a history of prolonged apnoea suggests pseudocholinesterase deficiency (see Chapter 4), and an unexplained death suggests malignant hyperpyrexia (see Chapter 4). Elective surgery should be postponed if any conditions are identified while the patient is being investigated appropriately. In the emergency situation, anaesthesia must be adjusted accordingly, for example by avoiding triggering drugs in a patient with a potential or actual family history of malignant hyperpyrexia.

Drug history and allergies

Identify all medications, both prescribed and over the counter (OTC), including complementary and alternative medicines. Patients will often forget to mention the oral contraceptive pill (OCP) and hormone replacement therapy (HRT) unless specifically asked. On the whole, the number of medications patients take rises with age. Many commonly prescribed drugs such as angiotensin converting enzyme inhibitors (ACE-I) can have important effects during anaesthesia. These can be identified by consulting a current British National Formulary (BNF) [2.2]. Allergies to drugs, latex, topical preparations (e.g. iodine), adhesive dressings and foodstuffs should be noted.

Social history

- *Smoking:* ascertain the amount of tobacco smoked. This is usually calculated as the number of pack-years: number of packs smoked each day multiplied by the number of years smoked. This gives an idea of the total amount smoked and allows comparison between individuals. In the long term, smoking causes chronic lung disease and carcinoma but it also has a number of other important effects relevant to the perioperative period. It produces carbon monoxide, which combines with haemoglobin and reduces oxygen carriage, and nicotine, which stimulates the sympathetic nervous system causing tachycardia, hypertension and coronary artery narrowing. Ciliary function is impaired, increasing the risk of postoperative chest infections. Stopping smoking before anaesthesia reduces the risk of perioperative complications – the further in advance, the better. As a guide, stopping for eight weeks improves the airways; for two weeks reduces airway irritability and for as little as 24 hours before anaesthesia decreases carboxyhaemoglobin levels. Help and advice should be available at the preoperative assessment clinic.
- *Alcohol:* this is measured as units consumed per week; >50 units/week causes induction of liver enzymes and tolerance to anaesthetic drugs. The risk of alcohol withdrawal syndrome postoperatively must be considered.
- *Drugs:* ask specifically about the use of drugs for recreational purposes, including type, frequency and route of administration. This group of patients is at risk of infection with hepatitis B and human immunodeficiency virus (HIV). There can be difficulty with venous access following intravenous drug abuse due to widespread thrombosis of veins. Withdrawal syndromes can occur postoperatively.
- *Pregnancy:* the date of the last menstrual period should be noted in all women of child-bearing age. The anaesthetist may be the only person in theatre able to give this information if X-rays are required. Anaesthesia increases the risk of inducing a spontaneous abortion in early pregnancy. There is an increased risk of regurgitation and aspiration in late pregnancy. Elective surgery is best postponed until after delivery.

Assessing the risk of postoperative nausea and vomiting

A significant proportion of patients experience postoperative nausea and vomiting (PONV), the frequency ranging from 25% to 80% in different patient groups. This has many adverse consequences including increased patient anxiety and dissatisfaction, increased pain, risk of aspiration, wound dehiscence and potential delayed discharge after day-case surgery. It is therefore useful to try and identify those at greatest risk to plan management when they present for surgery. There are four main independent risk factors that can help to predict a patient's likelihood of experiencing PONV:

- female;
- a non-smoker;
- previous history of PONV or motion sickness;
- using opioids as part of the anaesthetic technique.

The incidence of PONV increases with the number of risk factors and is approximately 10%, 20%, 40%, 60% and 80% in patients with zero, one, two, three or four risk factors respectively. A scoring system that allocates one point for each of the four risk factors listed above has been devised (the Apfel score) to try to stratify an individual patient's risk of PONV and guide prophylaxis. Patients who score:

- 0 or 1 points have a low risk of PONV and should not routinely receive antiemetics;
- 2 or more points have a high risk of PONV and should receive combination therapy (use drugs with different modes of action).

For patients with two or more risk factors, consideration should also be given to altering the anaesthetic technique to one associated with a lower incidence of PONV, for example a regional anaesthetic technique, general anaesthesia with total intravenous anaesthesia (TIVA), avoiding opioids where possible.

The examination

This concentrates on the cardiovascular and respiratory systems; the remaining systems are examined if problems relevant to anaesthesia have been identified in the history. At the end of the examination, the patient's airway is assessed to try and identify any potential problems. If a regional anaesthetic is planned, the appropriate anatomy (for example, lumbar spine for central neural block) is examined.

Cardiovascular system

Examine specifically for signs of:

- arrhythmias;
- heart failure;
- hypertension;
- valvular heart disease;
- peripheral vascular disease.

Don't forget to inspect the peripheral veins to identify any potential problems with intravenous (IV) access.

Respiratory system

Examine specifically for signs of:

- respiratory failure;
- impaired ventilation;
- collapse, consolidation, pleural effusion;
- additional or absent breath sounds.

Nervous system

Chronic disease of the peripheral and central nervous systems should be identified and any evidence of peripheral neuropathy, motor or sensory, recorded to ensure that any abnormalities postoperatively are not attributed to injury intraoperatively. It must be remembered that some disorders will affect the cardiovascular and respiratory systems, for example dystrophia myotonica and multiple sclerosis.

Musculoskeletal system

Note any restriction of movement and deformity if a patient has connective tissue disorders. Patients suffering from chronic rheumatoid disease frequently have a reduced muscle mass, peripheral neuropathies and pulmonary involvement. Particular attention should be paid to the patient's cervical spine and temporomandibular joints (see later).

The airway

The airway of all patients must be assessed, in order to try to predict those patients who may be difficult to intubate.

Observe the patient's anatomy, looking specifically for:

- limitation of mouth opening;
- a receding mandible;
- position, number and health of teeth;
- size of the tongue;
- soft tissue swelling at the front of the neck;
- deviation of the larynx or trachea;
- limitations in flexion and extension of the cervical spine.

Finding any of these suggests that intubation may be more difficult. However, it must be remembered that all of these are subjective.

Some simple bedside tests can also be performed.

- *Mallampati criteria:* the patient, sitting upright, is asked to open their mouth and maximally protrude their tongue. The view of the pharyngeal structures is noted and graded I–IV (Figure 2.1). Grades III and IV suggest difficult intubation.
- *Thyromental distance:* with the head fully extended on the neck, the distance between the bony point of the chin and the prominence of the thyroid cartilage is measured (Figure 2.2). A distance of less than 7 cm suggests difficult intubation.
- *Calder test:* the patient is asked to protrude the mandible as far as possible. The lower incisors will either lie anterior to, aligned with or posterior to the upper incisors. The latter two suggest reduced view at laryngoscopy.
- *Wilson score:* increasing weight, a reduction in head and neck movement, reduced mouth opening and the presence of a receding mandible or buck teeth all predispose to increased difficulty with intubation.

None of these tests, alone or in combination, will predict all difficult intubations. A Mallampati grade III or IV with a thyromental distance of <7 cm will predict 80% of difficult intubations. If problems are anticipated, anaesthesia should be planned accordingly. If intubation proves to be difficult, it must be recorded in a prominent place in the patient's notes and the patient informed.

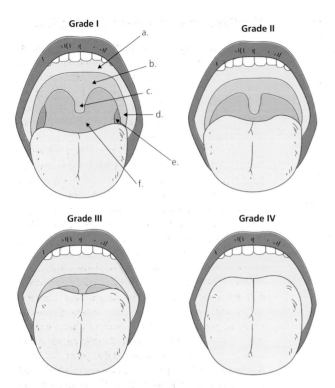

Figure 2.1 The pharyngeal structures seen during the Mallampati assessment. Grade I: Hard palate (a), soft palate (b), uvula (c), fauces (d), tonsillar pillars (e) and posterior pharyngeal wall (f) are visible. Grade II: Hard palate, soft palate, uvula, fauces and posterior pharyngeal wall visible. Grade III: Hard palate, soft palate and base of uvula visible. Grade IV: Only hard palate visible.

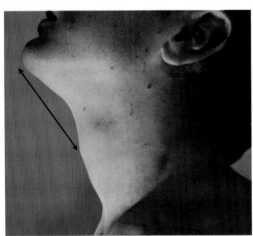

Figure 2.2 The thyromental distance.

Investigations

There is little evidence to support 'routine' investigations, and so an investigation should only be ordered if the result would affect the patient's management. In general, the type and number of investigations depend on the patient's age, the nature and severity of their comorbidities and the surgery planned. A synopsis of the current guidelines for *patients with no evidence of concurrent disease* (ASA 1, see later) is shown in Table 2.1. For each age group and grade of surgery, the upper entry shows 'tests recommended' and the lower entry 'tests to be considered' (depending on patient characteristics). Dipstick urinalysis need only be performed in symptomatic individuals.

Additional investigations

The following is a guide for when to request some of the common preoperative investigations. Again, the need for these will depend on the grade of surgery and the age of the patient.

Further information on preoperative tests can be found in Clinical Guideline 3, published by NICE [2.3].

- *Urea and electrolytes:* patients taking digoxin, diuretics or steroids and those with diabetes, renal disease, vomiting, diarrhoea.
- *Liver function tests:* known hepatic disease, a history of a high alcohol intake (>50 units/week), metastatic disease or evidence of malnutrition.
- *Blood sugar:* diabetics, severe peripheral arterial disease or taking long-term steroids.

- *Electrocardiogram:* hypertensive, with symptoms or signs of ischaemic heart disease, a cardiac arrhythmia or diabetics >40 years of age.
- *Chest X-ray:* symptoms or signs of cardiac or respiratory disease, or suspected or known malignancy, where thoracic surgery is planned, or in those from areas of endemic tuberculosis who have not had a chest X-ray in the last year.
- *Pulmonary function tests:* dyspnoea on mild exertion, COPD or asthma. Measure peak expiratory flow rate (PEFR), forced expiratory volume in 1 second (FEV_1) and FVC. Patients who are dyspnoeic or cyanosed at rest, found to have an $FEV_1 < 60\%$ predicted or are to have thoracic surgery should also have arterial blood gas analysed while breathing air.
- *Coagulation screen:* anticoagulant therapy, a history of a bleeding diatheses, or a history of liver disease or jaundice.
- *Sickle cell screen (sickledex):* a family history of sickle cell disease or where ethnicity increases the risk of sickle cell disease. If positive, electrophoresis will be required for definitive diagnosis.
- *Cervical spine X-ray:* rheumatoid arthritis, a history of major trauma or surgery to the neck, or when difficult intubation is predicted.

Cardiopulmonary exercise testing

Cardiopulmonary exercise (CPX) testing objectively determines each patient's ability to increase oxygen delivery to the tissues under controlled conditions and allows a preoperative assessment of their fitness. Consequently, high-risk patients can be identified allowing appropriate preparation to be made for their perioperative management.

To perform a CPX test, patients exercise using a bicycle ergometer, against an increasing resistance (like peddling uphill) while breathing through a mouthpiece (Figure 2.3). The volume and composition of inhaled and exhaled gases are monitored and analysed to determine oxygen consumption (VO_2, mL/min/kg), carbon dioxide production (VCO_2, mL/min/kg), respiratory rate, tidal volume and minute ventilation. The patient's peripheral oxygen saturation (SpO_2) and ECG are also usually monitored. The principle of the test is that, during exercise, VO_2 is the same as VCO_2. As the intensity of exercise increases, a point is reached where oxygen delivery can no longer meet metabolic demand and anaerobic metabolism starts. At this point, CO_2 production exceeds oxygen consumption; this is termed the anaerobic threshold (AT). If the intensity of exercise increases further, the oxygen consumption

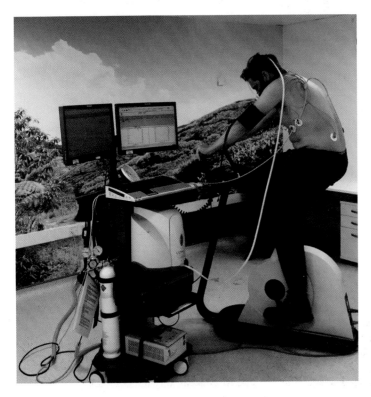

Figure 2.3 Cardiopulmonary exercise test taking place.

Table 2.3 Anaerobic threshold (AT) values used to predict risk and the need for an increased level of care postoperatively.

Value	Risk and level of care
AT >14 mL/min/kg	No specific risk, ward-based care
AT 11–14 mL/min/kg	Low risk, requires HDU care postoperatively
AT <11 mL/min/kg	High risk, requires ITU care postoperatively
Basal oxygen consumption	3.5 mL/kg/min

HDU, high dependency unit; ITU, intensive therapy unit.

will eventually plateau (VO_2 max). This equates to the peak aerobic capacity. Many assessments of fitness measure the AT as it occurs before VO_2 max, is more easily achieved by the elderly and is less influenced by patient motivation. The lower the AT, the less cardiopulmonary reserve the patient has and the greater risk of postoperative morbidity and mortality. Table 2.3 shows values that have been used to predict risk and the need for an increased level of care postoperatively.

Unfortunately, not all patients can be assessed in this way; for example, those with severe musculoskeletal dysfunction may not be able to exercise to their anaerobic threshold. In such circumstances further investigations will be required. The most readily available method of non-invasive assessment of cardiac function in patients is some type of echocardiography (see later). See also the American College of Cardiology/American Heart Association guidelines [2.4].

Echocardiography

This is a useful tool to assess many aspects of cardiac function in a number of diseases. In patients with heart failure or following a myocardial infarction, left ventricular function can be assessed by calculating the ejection fraction, observing the strength of contractility and looking for regional wall motion abnormalities caused by coronary artery disease. In patients with chronic pulmonary disease, the right ventricular function and pulmonary artery pressures can be assessed. In patients with aortic stenosis, the valve (aperture) area can be measured and the pressure gradient across the valve, which is a good indication of the severity of the disease, can be calculated. In patients with newly diagnosed atrial fibrillation, the presence of any intra-atrial blood clots can be identified. All of

these things are assessed with the patient at rest and so do not give any indication of what happens when metabolic demand is increased. It is possible to simulate exercise, and hence the conditions a patient may encounter during anaesthesia or after surgery. This is often achieved by administering an inotrope, such as dobutamine, which increases heart rate and myocardial work while any changes in myocardial performance are monitored (dobutamine stress echocardiography). This is particularly useful for assessing cardiac function in patients whose exercise ability is limited, for instance by severe osteoarthritis.

Medical referral

Patients with significant medical (or surgical) comorbidities should be identified in the preoperative assessment clinic, not on the day of admission, to allow time for adequate investigation and management. Clearly, a wide spectrum of conditions exists; the following are examples of some of the more commonly encountered that may need specialist advice.

Cardiovascular disease

- Untreated or poorly controlled hypertension or heart failure.
- Symptomatic ischaemic heart disease, despite treatment (unstable angina).
- Arrhythmias: uncontrolled atrial fibrillation, paroxysmal supraventricular tachycardia, and second- and third-degree heart block.
- Symptomatic or newly diagnosed valvular heart disease, or congenital heart disease.

Respiratory disease

- COPD, particularly if dyspnoeic at rest.
- Bronchiectasis.
- Asthmatics who are unstable, taking oral steroids or have a $FEV_1 < 60\%$ predicted.

Endocrine disorders

- Insulin-dependent and non-insulin-dependent diabetics who have ketonuria, glycosylated Hb (HbA1c) >10% or a random blood sugar >12 mmol/L. Local policy will dictate referral of stable diabetics for perioperative management.
- Hypo- or hyperthyroidism symptomatic on current treatment.
- Cushing's or Addison's disease.
- Hypopituitarism.

Renal disease

- Chronic renal failure.
- Patients undergoing renal replacement therapy.

Haematological disorders

- Bleeding diatheses, for example haemophilia, thrombocytopenia.
- Therapeutic anticoagulation.
- Haemoglobinopathies.
- Polycythaemia.
- Haemolytic anaemias.
- Leukaemias.

The obese patient

The commonest method of identifying overweight and obese patients is by calculation of their body mass index (BMI), which is expressed as:

$$Weight(kg)/\left[height(m)\right]^2$$

This is then used to divide people into different categories (Table 2.4).

However, there are recognized problems when relying on BMI alone as it does not differentiate between weight due to fat and that due to muscle. The latter is denser and heavily muscled individuals can appear to be overweight or even obese despite low amounts of total body fat. Furthermore, BMI does not provide any information about the distribution of fat within the body.

An alternative assessment, which does factor in fat distribution, is to calculate a patient's waist/height ratio. Central adiposity ('apple' body shape), where a higher proportion of fat surrounds the intra-abdominal viscera, is associated with a greater risk to health than peripheral adiposity ('pear' body shape). A waist/height ratio of >0.55 is associated with an increased risk to health. On balance, it is probably best to use both assessments to identify those at risk of obesity-related ill health.

The current guidelines from the Society for Obesity and Bariatric Anaesthesia (SOBA) [2.5] and the AAGBI [2.6] recommend more detailed assessment of sleep-disordered breathing and risk of venous thromboembolism (VTE) in obese patients. All patients with a BMI >35 should be screened for obstructive sleep apnoea (OSA) using the STOP-BANG tool (Table 2.5). A score of >5 indicates a risk of the patient having significant OSA which is associated with a higher incidence of difficult intubation, postoperative pulmonary and cardiovascular complications, increased intensive care unit admissions and a greater duration of hospital stay. The risk of complications is highest in patients previously undiagnosed with OSA or not using nocturnal continuous positive airway pressure (CPAP). Along with specific assessment of their cardiorespiratory system, this will guide further investigations and indicate the need for additional perioperative monitoring and support.

Cardiovascular system

Hypertension, ischaemic heart disease, atrial fibrillation, hyperlipidaemia and heart failure are commoner in obese patients. Although the history and examination may reveal signs and symptoms of cardiac disease, immobility often limits the patient's exercise tolerance and symptoms are not evident. A lower threshold should be used for requesting a 12-lead ECG and a stress echocardiogram may be indicated for patients who are unable to exercise sufficiently.

Respiratory system

A careful history should be taken of dyspnoea, exercise tolerance and OSA. Pulse oximetry can easily be carried out in the preoperative clinic and a supine $SpO_2 < 95\%$

Table 2.4 World Health Organization classification of obesity based on body mass index (BMI).

Category	BMI
Underweight	<18.5
Normal	18.5–24.9
Overweight	25.0–29.9
Obese 1	30.0–34.9
Obese 2	35.0–39.9
Obese 3 (morbidly obese)	>40

Table 2.5 STOP-BANG tool used to screen for sleep apnoea.

S	**S**noring. Do you snore loudly (louder than talking or heard through a closed door)?
T	**T**ired. Do you often feel tired or sleepy during the daytime?
O	**O**bserved. Has anyone observed you stop breathing during sleep?
P	Blood **P**ressure. Do you have or are you being treated for high blood pressure?
B	**B**MI >35 kg/m²
A	**A**ge >50 years
N	**N**eck. Circumference >43 cm (17 in) in males, >41 cm (16 in) in females
G	**G**ender: male

Each positive finding scores 1 point and the total is summed to give the STOP-BANG score.

Table 2.6 Cardiorespiratory warning signs in obese patients.

- Poor functional capacity
- An abnormal ECG; LV hypertrophy or strain, right axis deviation, RBBB, P pulmonale, inferior T waves
- Uncontrolled blood pressure or ischaemic heart disease
- $SpO_2 < 95\%$ on air
- Poorly controlled asthma or COPD
- Previous DVT or pulmonary embolus (PE)
- STOP-BANG score >5 (see Table 2.5)

COPD, chronic obstructive pulmonary disease; DVT, deep vein thrombosis; ECG, electrocardiogram; LV, left ventricular; PE, pulmonary embolism; RBBB, right bundle branch block.

on room air suggests that further investigations or referral to a respiratory physician are appropriate. Morbidly obese patients with asthma or COPD are at even greater risk of perioperative respiratory complications. Wheeze in obese patients may be due to airway closure rather than asthma; in up to 50% of patients this resolves with weight loss. Pulmonary function tests before and after bronchodilator therapy may be useful in differentiation between the two conditions.

A summary of cardiorespiratory warning signs is given in Table 2.6. In patients who have **any** of the findings in Table 2.6, consideration must be given to:

- arterial blood gas analysis and sleep studies;
- preoperative CPAP;
- echocardiography;
- cardiorespiratory referral;
- anaesthesia (perioperative care) by a team who are experienced in managing obese patients;
- postoperative care in a high-dependency unit (HDU) if undergoing major surgery.

Metabolic and gastrointestinal systems

Morbidly obese patients have a high incidence of diabetes mellitus. All patients should be questioned about symptoms of diabetes and have appropriate investigations if symptomatic. Those known to be diabetic should be assessed for the adequacy of glucose control, for example HbA1c, and also for the presence of complications, especially coronary artery disease, diabetic nephropathy and autonomic dysfunction. Improved perioperative glucose control may help reduce complications such as wound infections or the development of keto- or lactic acidosis. Ask about symptoms of acid reflux; appropriate antacid prophylaxis may be indicated preoperatively.

Other issues

Preoperative assessment several weeks prior to planned surgery will allow the opportunity to optimize the patient's medical comorbidities, plan for anaesthesia and arrange the appropriate level of postoperative care. Informed consent should be obtained with discussion of any specific increased risks related to anaesthesia (see later). Following full assessment and an explanation of the potential risks, some patients may reconsider whether or not to proceed with surgery.

Risks associated with anaesthesia and surgery

One of the questions most commonly asked of anaesthetists is 'What are the risks of having an anaesthetic?' The Royal College of Anaesthetists and the AAGBI have issued a guide for patients entitled *You and Your Anaesthetic* [2.7]. This divides the risks associated with anaesthesia and their frequency as follows.

Common (1 in 10 to 1 in 100)

These are not life threatening and can occur even when anaesthesia has apparently been uneventful. They include:

- bruising and soreness from attempts at IV access;
- sore throat;
- headache;
- dizziness;
- postoperative nausea and vomiting;
- itching;
- retention of urine.

Uncommon (1 in 1000)

These include:

- dental damage;
- chest infection;
- muscle pains;
- an existing condition worsening, such as myocardial infarction;
- awareness during general anaesthesia.

Rare (<1 in 10 000)

These include:

- allergy to the anaesthetic drugs;
- eye injury, particularly if in prone position;
- nerve damage;
- hypoxic brain injury;
- death.

In the United Kingdom, the Royal College of Anaesthetists quote a risk of 1 death per 100 000 anaesthetics in healthy individuals having non-emergency surgery [2.8]. This is based on the findings of the Confidential Enquiry into Perioperative Deaths (CEPOD 1987) which found an overall perioperative mortality of 0.7% in approximately 500 000 operations. Anaesthesia was judged *completely* responsible in only three cases – a primary mortality rate of 1:185 000 operations. Upon analysis of the deaths where anaesthesia contributed, the predominant factor was human error.

Clearly, anaesthesia itself is very safe, particularly in those patients who are otherwise well. Apart from human error, the most likely major risk is from an adverse drug reaction or drug interaction. However, anaesthesia rarely occurs in isolation and when the risks of the surgical procedure and those due to pre-existing disease are combined, the risks of morbidity and mortality are increased. Not surprisingly, a number of methods have been described to try to quantify these risks.

Risk indicators

The most widely used scale for estimating risk is the ASA classification of the patient's physical status. The patient is assigned to a category from one to five, depending on any physical disturbance caused by either the disease process for which surgery is being performed or any other pre-existing disease. It is relatively subjective, which leads to a degree of variability between scorers. Different studies have reported different mortalities for each grade. This is a result of differences in populations of patients, sample sizes, types of surgery being performed and the duration of patient monitoring postoperatively, for example deaths at 48 hours or at one week. However, patients placed in higher categories are at increased overall risk of perioperative mortality (Table 2.7).

The leading cause of death after surgery is myocardial infarction, and significant morbidity results from non-fatal infarction, particularly in patients with pre-existing heart disease. As well as the risks from pre-existing

Table 2.7 ASA physical status scale.

Class	Physical status	Absolute mortality (%)
I	A healthy patient with no organic or psychological disease process. The pathological process for which the operation is being performed is localized and causes no systemic upset	0–0.3
II	A patient with a mild-to-moderate systemic disease process, caused by the condition to be treated surgically or another pathological process, that does not limit the patient's activities in any way, e.g. treated hypertensive, stable diabetic. Patients aged >80 years are automatically placed in class II	0.3–1.4
III	A patient with severe systemic disease from any cause that imposes a definite functional limitation on activity, e.g. ischaemic heart disease, COPD	1.5–5.4
IV	A patient with a severe systemic disease that is a constant threat to life, e.g. unstable angina	7.8–25.9
V	A moribund patient unlikely to survive 24 hours with or without surgery	9.4–57.8
VI	A patient declared brain dead whose organs are being removed for transplantation	

Note: 'E' may be added to signify an emergency operation. COPD, chronic obstructive pulmonary disease.

cardiac disease, different operations also carry their own varying levels of inherent risks; for example, carpal tunnel decompression carries less risk than a hip replacement, which in turn carries less risk than aortic aneurysm surgery. Basically, this can be summarized as 'the sicker the patient and the bigger the operation, the greater the risk.'

Assessing patients as 'low risk' is no more of a guarantee that complications will not occur than 'high risk' means they will occur; it is only a guideline and indicator of probability. For patients who suffer a complication, the rate is 100%! Ultimately, the risk/benefit ratio must be considered for each individual patient. If a patient has a certain predicted risk of complications, an operation with the potential to offer only a small benefit may be deemed not worth the risk, whereas one with the potential to offer a large benefit may be undertaken. Clearly, this is a decision that can only be reached after careful and thorough discussion with a patient who has been given all the relevant information.

Improving preoperative preparation by optimizing the patient's physical status, adequately resuscitating those who require emergency surgery, appropriate intraoperative monitoring, and by providing suitable postoperative care in an appropriate level of critical care has been shown to further reduce patients' perioperative mortality.

Specific risks in extreme obesity

Although the majority of overweight and obese patients are relatively healthy and have risks similar to patients of normal weight, those with extreme obesity are at higher risk. The Obesity Surgery Mortality Risk Score (OS-MRS), although developed for patients undergoing bariatric surgery, may be useful in those undergoing non-bariatric surgery. The presence of each risk factor scores 1 point and the sum is used to calculate risk of mortality (Table 2.8).

Table 2.8 Obesity Surgery Mortality Risk Score.

Risk factor	Score
BMI >50 kg/m²	1
Male	1
Age >45 years	1
Hypertension	1
Risk factors for pulmonary embolism:	1
Previous VTE	
Vena caval filter	
Sleep-disordered breathing	
Pulmonary hypertension	
Risk of mortality	
0–1 point	0.2–0.3%
2–3 points	1.1–1.5%
4–5 points	2.4–3.0%

The presence of each risk factor scores 1 point.

Classification of operation

Traditionally, surgery was classified as being either elective or emergency. Recognizing that this was too imprecise, the National Confidential Enquiry into Perioperative Outcome and Death (NCEPOD) has identified four categories.

1 *Immediate:* to save life, limb or organ. Resuscitation is simultaneous with surgery. The target time to theatre is within minutes of the decision that surgery is necessary – for example, major trauma to the abdomen or thorax with uncontrolled haemorrhage, major neurovascular deficit, ruptured aortic aneurysm.

2 *Urgent:* acute onset or deterioration of a condition that threatens life, limb or organ. Surgery normally takes place when resuscitation is complete. Examples would be compound fracture, perforated viscus, cauda equina syndrome. This category is subdivided into:
  2A Target time to theatre within 6 hours of the decision to operate
  2B Target time to theatre within 24 hours of the decision to operate

3 *Expedited:* stable patient requiring early intervention. Condition not an immediate threat to life, limb or organ. Target time to theatre is within days of the decision to operate. Examples would be closed fracture, tendon injury, some tumour surgery.

4 *Elective:* surgery planned and booked in advance of admission to hospital. This category includes all conditions not covered in categories 1–3. Typical examples would be joint replacements, cholecystectomy, hernia repair.

All elective and the majority of expedited cases can be assessed as previously described. In urgent and emergency cases, this will not always be possible, but as much information as possible should be obtained about allergies, the patient's medical history, drugs taken regularly and previous anaesthetics. In the trauma patient, enquire about the mechanism of injury. This may give clues to unsuspected injuries. Details may only be available from relatives and/or the ambulance crew. The cardiovascular and respiratory systems should be examined and an assessment made of any potential difficulty with intubation. Investigations should only be ordered if they would directly affect the conduct of anaesthesia. When life or limb is at stake, there will be even less or no time for assessment. All emergency patients should be assumed to have a full stomach.

Prevention of venous thromboembolism

Up to 25 000 patients die each year in the UK as a result of a hospital-acquired VTE. It is now a requirement that all patients admitted to hospital are assessed for their risk of developing a VTE and appropriate preventative measures applied. Surgical patients and patients with trauma are at increased risk of VTE with:

- a total anaesthetic and surgical time >90 minutes;
- surgery to the pelvis or lower limb and the total anaesthetic and surgical time >60 minutes;
- an acute surgical admission with inflammatory or intra-abdominal condition;
- an expected reduction in mobility.

Further non-surgical factors increase the risk of VTE:

- active cancer or treatment for cancer;
- age >60 years;
- critical care admission;
- dehydration;
- known thrombophilia;
- BMI >30 kg/m^2;
- one or more significant medical comorbidities (for example, heart disease, respiratory disease, endocrine or metabolic disorders);
- personal or first-degree relative with a history of VTE;
- use of HRT;
- use of oestrogen-containing contraceptive;
- varicose veins with phlebitis.

Patients must also be assessed for their risk of bleeding:

- active bleeding;
- acquired coagulopathy (for example, liver failure);
- concurrent anticoagulation;
- epidural, spinal anaesthesia (or lumbar puncture) within the last 4 hours or expected within 12 hours;
- acute stroke;
- thrombocytopenia;
- uncontrolled hypertension (>230/120 mmHg);
- untreated bleeding disorders (for example, haemophilia).

Where the risks of VTE exceed the risks of bleeding, VTE prophylaxis should be used. The method employed will depend upon the type and site of surgery and may be mechanical (for example, antiembolism stockings, pneumatic calf compression) or pharmacological (for example, heparin, fondiparinux or rivaroxaban). All patients should be reassessed 24 hours after admission to identify any clinical changes, to ensure that the method chosen has been implemented and to identify any adverse effects.

Obtaining informed consent

What is consent?

Consent is an agreement by the patient to undergo a specific procedure. Even though the doctor will advise on what is required, it is only the patient who can make the decision to undergo the procedure. Although the need for consent is often thought of as applying to surgery, it is in fact required for any breach of a patient's personal integrity, including examination, performing investigations and giving an anaesthetic. Touching a patient without consent may lead to a claim of battery. Consent may be explicit or expressed, for example when a person agrees, either verbally or in writing. Consent can also be implied as indicated by an informed patient's behaviour, but this form of consent only has validity if the patient genuinely knows and understands what is being proposed. An example would be a patient voluntarily holding an arm out for a blood test after an explanation of why the test is needed. Whatever form of consent is obtained, providing sufficient, accurate information is essential. When patients do not know what is proposed or are unaware that they can refuse, they have not given consent. In medicine, when obtaining consent for an operation or invasive procedure, it is written, explicit consent that is most commonly used.

All people aged 16 years and over are presumed, in law, to have the capacity to consent to treatment unless there is evidence to the contrary. Suffering from a mental disorder or impairment does not automatically mean lack of competence [2.9]. Some patients who would normally be considered competent may be temporarily incapable of giving valid consent due to intoxication from drugs or alcohol, severe pain or shock. A decision that appears to be irrational or unjustified should not be taken as evidence that the individual lacks the mental capacity to make that decision.

For a patient to have the capacity to give valid consent, there are five prerequisites. They should:

- understand what is being proposed, its purpose and why it is being proposed;
- understand the benefits, risks and any alternatives;

- understand the consequences of not receiving what is being proposed;
- retain the information long enough to arrive at a decision;
- be able to communicate their decision.

The decision the patient makes does not have to appear sensible or rational to anybody else. However, every effort must be made to ensure that a highly irrational decision is not the result of a lack of information or misinterpretation of the information given. It may, of course, also indicate that the patient is suffering from a mental illness. Determining capacity in these circumstances is probably best placed in the hands of the courts.

Refusal of treatment by a competent adult is legally binding (except where the law states otherwise, for example under mental health legislation), even if refusal is likely to lead to the patient's death (for example, a Jehovah's Witness refusing a blood transfusion). Although a patient can refuse treatment or choose a less than optimal option, they cannot insist on a treatment that has not been offered.

What do I have to tell the patient?

Although the anaesthetist is the best judge of the type of anaesthetic for each individual, where there is a choice, patients should be given an explanation along with the associated risks and benefits of the options. Recent legal rulings have made it clear that the assessment of whether a risk is material cannot be reduced to percentages and it cannot be left to the clinician to determine what to disclose. The doctor is under a duty to take reasonable care to ensure that the patient is aware of any material risks involved in proposed treatment, and of reasonable alternatives. A risk is 'material' if a reasonable person in the patient's position would be likely to attach significance to it, or if the doctor is or should reasonably be aware that their patient would be likely to attach significance to it [2.10]. A balance is required between listening to what the patient wants and providing enough information in terms they can understand; they do not have to ask specific questions. However, if they express concerns, these must be explored and answered providing enough information, in terms that the patient can understand, in order that the patient's decisions are informed. It has been suggested that even a risk as small as 0.01% of a serious event warrants discussion during the consent process (see Further information). Doctors can no longer rely on the practice of other doctors as a defence when disputes over consent are judged in court (the Bolam principle).

Typical information regarding anaesthesia may be:

- the environment of the anaesthetic room and who patients will meet, particularly if medical students or other healthcare professionals in training will be present;
- the need for intravenous access and IV infusion (a drip);
- the need for, and type of, any invasive monitoring;
- what to expect during a regional technique;
- being conscious throughout surgery if a regional technique alone is used and what they may hear;
- preoxygenation;
- use of cricoid pressure;
- induction of anaesthesia: although most commonly intravenous, occasionally it may be by inhalation;
- where they will 'wake up' – this is usually the recovery unit, but after some surgery it may be in a critical care area (in these circumstances the patient should be given the opportunity to visit the unit a few days before and meet some of the staff);
- numbness and loss of movement after regional anaesthesia;
- the possibility of drains, catheters and drips – patients may misinterpret their presence as indicating unexpected problems;
- the possibility of a need for blood transfusion;
- postoperative pain control, particularly if it requires their cooperation – for example, a patient-controlled analgesia device (see Chapter 8);
- information on risks associated with the anaesthetic technique (see earlier).

Most patients will want to know the latest time that they can eat and drink before surgery, if they should take their medications as normal and how they will manage without a drink. The Royal College of Anaesthetists and AAGBI recommend that in patients with normal gastric emptying, the evidence is that clear fluids empty rapidly and consequently day cases and inpatients can be allowed clear fluids for up to 2 hours before anaesthesia. This will not include patients with conditions that delay gastric emptying, for example, trauma, pain or gastrointestinal disease, and where there is use of opioid drugs. The evidence for solids is less clear but consensus opinion is a period of 6 hours fasting after a light meal; milk or drinks containing milk are acceptable. Some will expect or request a premed and in these circumstances, the approximate timing, route of administration and likely effects should be discussed. Finally, before leaving, ask if the patient has any questions or wants anything clarifying further.

Having given the patient the information considered relevant to them, they must have sufficient time to think it through and come to a decision. Consequently, the process of informed consent cannot occur solely at the point of admission or, even worse, in the anaesthetic room immediately before surgery! As a result, the process usually starts in the preoperative assessment clinic when information is often given to the patient in the form of a leaflet, such as *You and Your Anaesthetic*, published jointly by the Royal College of Anaesthetists and the AAGBI [2.7].

Who should obtain consent?

From the above, it is clear that the individual seeking consent must be able to provide all the necessary information for the patient and to answer the patient's questions. This will require the individual to be trained in, and familiar with, the procedure for which consent is sought, and is best done by a senior clinician or the person who is to perform the procedure. Complex problems may require a multidisciplinary approach to obtaining consent.

Where there has been a significant interval between obtaining consent for the procedure and the start of treatment, or if new information is available, consent should be reaffirmed. The aim is to provide any new information and allow patients the opportunity to ask questions and to review their decision. This process may be delegated to a doctor who is trained, qualified and familiar with the procedure, who can answer the patient's questions.

The issues around consent in children and adults who lack capacity are more complex. More information is available in the document *Consent for Anaesthesia*, published by the AAGBI [2.11].

What constitutes evidence of consent?

Most patients will be asked to sign a consent form before undergoing a procedure. However, there is no legal requirement for this before anaesthesia or surgery (or anything else). Consent may be given verbally and this is often the case for anaesthesia; however, it is recommended that a written record of the content of the conversation be made in the patient's case notes.

What about an unconscious patient?

This usually arises in the emergency situation, for example a patient with a severe head injury. Asking a relative or other individual to sign a consent form for surgery on the patient's behalf is not appropriate, as no one can give consent on behalf of another adult. Under these circumstances, if an intervention is required to save a patient's life or avoid significant deterioration in their health before they will regain capacity to consent, medical staff are required to act 'in the patient's best interests'. This will mean taking into account not only the benefits of the proposed treatment but also personal and social factors. Such information may necessitate a discussion with relatives, and the opportunity should be used to inform them of the proposed treatment and the rationale for it. Where there is clear evidence of a valid advance refusal by an adult of a particular treatment (such as a refusal of blood by a Jehovah's Witness) then that treatment must not be given. If a patient has appointed a welfare attorney or there is a court-appointed deputy or guardian, where practicable this individual must be consulted about any proposed treatment.

The basis for any decision and how it is in the patient's best interests must be clearly documented in the patient's notes. Where treatment decisions are complex or not clear-cut, it is advisable, although not a legal requirement, to obtain and document independent medical advice.

For more detail on consent, the reader is strongly encouraged to refer to the *Consent Tool Kit*, published by the British Medical Association [2.12] and Department of Health guidelines [2.13].

FURTHER INFORMATION

Agnew N. Preoperative cardiopulmonary exercise testing. *Continuing Education in Anaesthesia, Critical Care and Pain* 2010; **10**(2): 33–37.

Dhesi JK, Swart M. Specialist pre-operative assessment clinics. *Anaesthesia* 2016; **71**(Suppl. 1): 3–8.

Janssen NB, Oort F, Fockens P, *et al.* Under what conditions do patients want to be informed about their risk of a complication? A vignette study. *Journal of Medical Ethics* 2009; **35**: 276–282.

Nadella V, Howell SJ. Hypertension: pathophysiology and perioperative implications. *BJA Education* 2015; **15**(6): 275–279.

Nightingale CE, Margarson MP, Shearer E, *et al.* Perioperative management of the obese surgical patient. *Anaesthesia* 2015; **70**: 859–876.

Wolters U, Wolf T, Stutzer H, Schroder T. ASA classification and perioperative variables as predictors of postoperative outcome. *British Journal of Anaesthesia* 1996; **77**: 217–222.

[2.1] www.aagbi.org/publications/guidelines/docs/preop2010.pdf
Preoperative assessment and patient preparation. The role of the anaesthetist. Association of Anaesthetists of Great Britain and Ireland. November 2010.

[2.2] www.medicinescomplete.com/mc/bnf/current/
The current British National Formulary (BNF) online.

[2.3] http://guidance.nice.org.uk/CG3/NICEGuidance/pdf/English
National Institute for Health and Care Excellence (NICE) guidance on preoperative tests. June 2003.

[2.4] http://content.onlinejacc.org/article.aspx?articleid=1893784
ACC/AHA 2014 Guideline on Perioperative Cardiovascular Evaluation for Noncardiac Surgery. A Report of the American College of Cardiology/American Heart Association Task Force on Practice Guidelines.

[2.5] http://sobauk.co.uk
Society for Obesity and Bariatric Anaesthesia web site. Up-to-date guidelines on the anaesthetic management of obese patients.

[2.6] http://onlinelibrary.wiley.com/enhanced/doi/10.1111/anae.13101/
Perioperative management of the obese surgical patient 2015. Association of Anaesthetists of Great Britain and Ireland.

[2.7] www.rcoa.ac.uk/document-store/you-and-your-anaesthetic
Patient information guides from the Association of Anaesthetists of Great Britain and Ireland and Royal College of Anaesthetists.

[2.8] www.rcoa.ac.uk/system/files/PI-RISK15-DEATH-2013
Patient information from the Royal College of Anaesthetists: Risks associated with your anaesthetic – Section 15 Death or brain damage.

[2.9] www.legislation.gov.uk/ukpga/2005/9/contents
Mental Capacity Act 2005. Department of Constitutional Affairs.

[2.10] www.supremecourt.uk/cases/uksc-2013-0136.html
Details of the High Court decision in the case of Montgomery v Lanarkshire Health Board.

[2.11] www.aagbi.org/publications/guidelines/docs/consent06.pdf
Consent for anaesthesia. Revised edition 2006. Association of Anaesthetists of Great Britain and Ireland.

[2.12] http://bma.org.uk/support-at-work/ethics/consent/consent-tool-kit
BMA consent tool kit.

[2.13] www.dh.gov.uk/en/Publicationsandstatistics/Publications/PublicationsPolicyAndGuidance/DH_103643
Department of Health (UK) guidance on consent. Second edition.

3

Anaesthetic equipment and monitoring

Learning objectives

After reading this chapter you should understand the principles of:

☐ How to use different types of airway equipment

☐ How gases and vapours are delivered to the patient

☐ The functions of the anaesthesia machine

☐ Mechanical ventilation

☐ The utility and limitations of devices commonly used to monitor the patient

Apply this knowledge when practising the following skills:

☐ Applying basic monitoring devices to a patient

☐ Interpreting pulse oximetry readings

☐ Interpreting the basic capnography waveform

Anaesthesia is a very practical specialty and, to practise safely, anaesthetists must be familiar with the equipment used. This ranges from the simple to the technical and its complexity is increasing relentlessly. The Medicines and Healthcare products Regulatory Agency (UK) (MHRA) ensures that all equipment and medicines meet appropriate standards of safety [3.1]. The following is an overview of the equipment and monitoring currently in use. No excuse is made for including very simple devices; these are often the most valuable but if used wrongly may endanger the patient's safety [3.2].

Clinical Anaesthesia: Lecture Notes, Fifth Edition. Matthew Gwinnutt and Carl Gwinnutt.
© 2017 John Wiley & Sons, Ltd. Published 2017 by John Wiley & Sons, Ltd.
Companion website: www.lecturenoteseries.com/anaesthesia

Airway equipment

The ability to ensure that a patient has a patent airway at all times is arguably the most important skill that an anaesthetist possesses. There is an ever-increasing range of airway conduits and equipment to aid their insertion available to the anaesthetist [3.3]. The safe and efficient use of the various devices relies on some common knowledge, for example of airway anatomy, but also skills unique to the equipment being used. It would be impossible to cover in detail all the currently available airway equipment, and unrealistic to expect someone to be skilled in the use of every device available. The important thing is to know when and how to use a selected range of devices well. The following is a description of most of the commonly available airway equipment; a description of the skills needed to use it safely and successfully is given in Chapter 5.

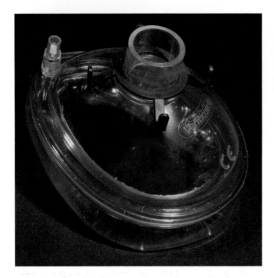

Figure 3.1 Plastic, disposable facemask.

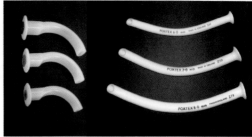

Figure 3.2 Oropharyngeal and nasopharyngeal airways.

Facemasks

These are designed to fit closely to the contours of the face and a gas-tight fit with the patient's face is achieved by an air-filled cuff around the edge. They are almost always single use and are made from transparent plastics, allowing visualization of vomit and misting during successful ventilation, making them popular for use during resuscitation (Figure 3.1).

Simple adjuncts

The oropharyngeal (Guedel) airway, and to a lesser extent the nasopharyngeal airway, are often used to help maintain the airway immediately after the induction of anaesthesia. However, their use does not guarantee a patent airway or offer any protection from airway soiling.

Oropharyngeal airway

These are curved plastic tubes, flattened in cross-section and flanged at the oral end (Figure 3.2). They lie over the tongue and prevent it from falling back into the pharynx. They are manufactured in a variety of sizes and are suitable for all patients, from neonates to large adults. The commonest sizes are 2–4, for small to large adults, respectively. The size required is estimated by comparing the airway length with the vertical distance between the patient's incisor teeth and the angle of the jaw.

Nasopharyngeal airway

These are round, malleable plastic tubes, bevelled at the pharyngeal end and flanged at the nasal end (Figure 3.2). They lie along the floor of the nose and curve round into the pharynx. They are sized according to their internal diameter in millimeters, and their length increases with the diameter. They are not commonly used in children, and sizes 6–8 mm in diameter are suitable for small to large adults, respectively. The correct size is estimated by comparing the airway diameter with that of the external nares.

Supraglottic airway (SGA) devices

Laryngeal mask airway (LMA)

This was the original supraglottic airway device and, as its name suggests, it consists of a 'mask' that sits over the laryngeal opening. This is attached to a tube that protrudes from the mouth and connects directly to the anaesthetic breathing system. Around the perimeter of the mask is an inflatable cuff that helps to stabilize it and creates a seal around the laryngeal inlet. LMAs are suitable for use in all patients, from neonates to adults, as they are produced in a variety of sizes. The most commonly used in female and male adults are sizes 3, 4 and 5. They were originally designed for use in spontaneously breathing patients. However, it is possible to ventilate patients via a LMA but care must be taken when doing this to avoid high inflation pressures, otherwise leakage occurs past the cuff, reducing ventilation and potentially causing gastric inflation. The original LMA (or classic LMA) is a reusable device requiring sterilization between each patient. In common with most airway equipment, these have been replaced with ones that are single use (Figure 3.3a) following concerns about the risk of prion disease (tissue spongiform encephalopathy) transmission.

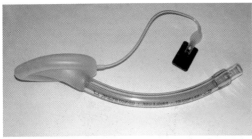

(a)

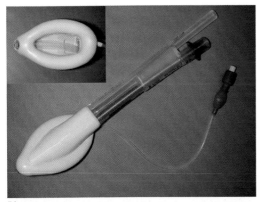

(b)

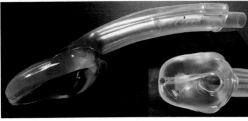

(c)

Figure 3.3 Supraglottic airway devices. (a) Disposable LMA. (b) LMA Pro-Seal™. (c) i-gel™.

There have been a number of modifications to the LMA.

- A version with a more flexible and reinforced tube. This is useful in maxillofacial or ear, nose and throat surgery as it allows the tube part to be flexed and directed out of the surgeon's way without kinking and occlusion of the lumen.
- The LMA Pro-Seal™ (Figure 3.3b). This has an additional posterior cuff to improve the seal between mask and larynx, and reduce leak when the patient is ventilated. It also has a secondary tube to allow drainage of gastric contents.

- The i-gel™ (Figure 3.3c). This uses a solid, highly malleable, gel-like material contoured to fit the perilaryngeal anatomy in place of the traditional inflatable cuff. It also features a narrow suction channel for aspiration of gastric contents and reinforcing plastic around the main tube which functions as a 'bite-block'. It is single use.

Tracheal tubes

These are manufactured from plastic (PVC), are single use to eliminate cross-infection, and are sized according to their internal diameter. They are available in a range of sizes at 0.5 mm diameter intervals, making them suitable for use in all patients from neonates to adults, and are long enough to be used orally or nasally. A standard 15 mm connector is provided to allow connection to the breathing system (Figure 3.4a).

The tracheal tubes used during adult anaesthesia have an inflatable cuff to prevent leakage of anaesthetic gases back past the tube when positive pressure ventilation is used, and also to prevent aspiration of any foreign material into the lungs. The cuff is inflated by injecting air via a pilot tube, at the distal end of which is a one-way valve to prevent deflation and a small 'balloon' to indicate when the cuff is inflated. A variety of specialized tubes have been developed, examples of which are shown in Figure 3.4b–d.

- *Preformed tubes:* used during surgery on the head and neck. These can either be 'north' (towards the forehead) or 'south' (towards the chin) facing and are designed to take the connections and breathing system tubing away from the surgical field (e.g. south-facing RAE tube, Figure 3.4b).
- *Reinforced tubes:* used when a plain tube might kink and become obstructed, e.g. due to the positioning of the patient's head or as a result of surgical manipulation (Figure 3.4c).
- *Double-lumen tubes:* effectively two tubes welded together side by side, with one tube extending distally beyond the other. They are used during intrathoracic surgery, and allow the anaesthetist to ventilate one lung selectively, thereby allowing optimal surgical access to the non-ventilated hemithorax. They are described as 'left' or 'right' sided depending on which main bronchus the tip of the tube lies within (Figure 3.4d) (see Chapter 7).
- *Uncuffed tubes:* used in children up to approximately 8 years of age as the narrowing in the subglottic region provides a natural seal. (Specialized cuffed tubes for children below this age are used in some paediatric units.)

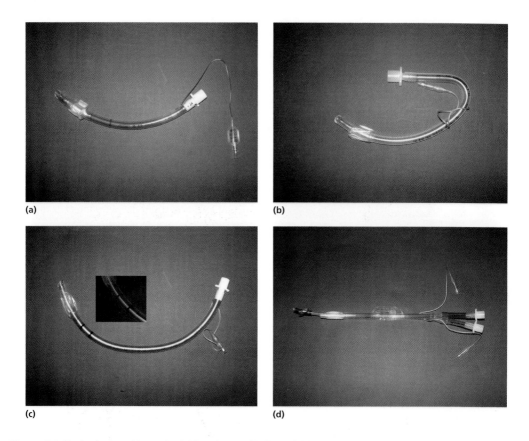

(a)

(b)

(c)

(d)

Figure 3.4 Tracheal tubes: (a) standard, (b) preformed (RAE tube), (c) reinforced tube, (d) double-lumen tube.

Laryngoscopes

Direct

These are the traditional laryngoscopes, designed to allow direct visualization of the larynx to facilitate the insertion of a tracheal tube. They consist of a blade with a light at the tip, attached to a handle that contains the batteries for the light. The most popular type in use is the curved blade designed by, and named after, Sir Robert Macintosh (Figure 3.5a). Different sized blades are available. There have been many developments in the design of this device, and one of the most successful is the McCoy blade (Figure 3.5b,c). This has a hinged tip operated by a lever adjacent to the handle that increases the elevation of the epiglottis to improve the view of the larynx. Occasionally, a straight-bladed laryngoscope may be used, such as the Magill blade.

Indirect

Recently, numerous devices have been developed that make use of advanced optics and electronics in order to overcome the difficulties when the larynx cannot be directly visualized using the laryngoscopes described above. The operator can visualize the larynx either by 'looking through' these devices or by having the image displayed on a separate screen. Some examples that highlight the different technologies used are included here.

- *Videolaryngoscopes*: there are several of these devices available from different manufacturers, for example the Glidescope®. A video camera and light source are placed within a single-use, curved blade (Figure 3.5d). The image is displayed on an adjacent screen and allows a better view of the larynx. Different sized and shaped blades are available allowing use in patients of all ages. A common pitfall of these devices is that despite a good view of the laryngeal inlet, difficulty is encountered passing a tracheal tube due to the exaggerated curvature of the laryngoscope blade. In order to overcome this problem, either a tracheal tube guide is incorporated into the laryngoscope blade or a curved stylet or bougie is used. These devices also have a role to play in

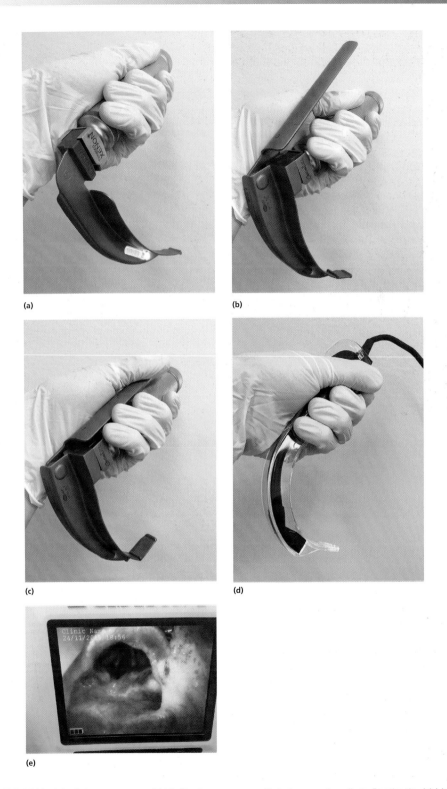

Figure 3.5 (a) Macintosh laryngoscope. (b) McCoy laryngoscope. Note lever on handle to flex the tip. (c) McCoy laryngoscope with tip flexed. (d) Glidescope® with view of larynx seen on screen.

training, as a supervisor can see what the student sees and offer advice and guidance to improve technique.

- *Fibreoptic bronchoscope* (Figure 3.6): a narrow diameter flexible bronchoscope that transmits the image from the tip of the scope via thousands of small diameter glass fibres to an eyepiece or display monitor. The tip is manoeuvrable from the handle to help guide the scope in the right direction, and there is a suction channel to remove any secretions from the airways. It can be used to guide a tracheal tube into position, and also is essential to check that a double-lumen tube is appropriately positioned. This procedure can be done with the patient awake, following suitable sedation and airway anaesthesia, or with the patient anaesthetized. Fibreoptic bronchoscopes need cleaning and sterilizing between patients.
- *Optical stylets* (Figure 3.7): very similar in principle to the flexible fibreoptic bronchoscope except that they are rigid, and only suitable for oral use in patients under general anaesthesia.

Tracheal tube introducers

These are usually 60 cm long and constructed of a malleable material that allows them to be bent into a gentle curve before being introduced, to be directed blindly behind the epiglottis into the trachea. They are rigid enough to allow a tracheal tube to be passed over them into the trachea.

Difficult airway trolley

Each operating theatre suite and intensive therapy unit (ITU) within a hospital will usually have a difficult airway trolley (Figure 3.8). Ideally, these are standardized (in terms of both equipment contained and layout) across the hospital and contain a selection of the airway equipment described above to allow the anaesthetist to deal with a difficult airway.

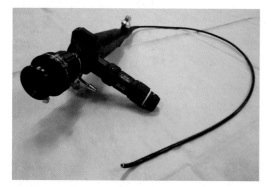

Figure 3.6 Fibreoptic bronchoscope.

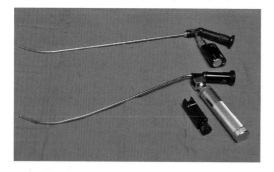

Figure 3.7 Optical stylets. Bonfils (*above*), Shikani (*below*). Source: McGuire and Younger (2010). Reproduced with permission of Oxford University Press.

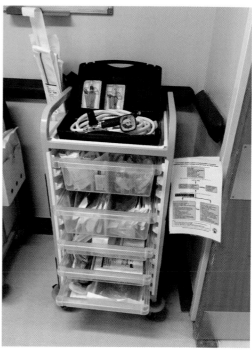

Figure 3.8 A typical difficult airway trolley.

The safe delivery of anaesthesia

Delivery of gases to the operating theatre

Most hospitals use a piped medical gas and vacuum system (PMGV) to distribute oxygen, nitrous oxide, medical air and vacuum. The pipelines' outlets act as self-closing sockets, each specifically configured, coloured and labelled for one gas. Oxygen, nitrous oxide and air are delivered to the anaesthetic room at a pressure of 400 kilopascals (kPa) (4 bar, 60 pounds per square inch (psi)). The gases (and vacuum) reach the anaesthetic machine via flexible reinforced hoses, colour-coded throughout their length (oxygen – white, nitrous oxide – blue, vacuum – yellow). These attach to the wall outlet via a gas-specific probe and to the anaesthetic machine via a gas-specific nut and union. Cylinders are used as reserves in case of pipeline failure.

The gas content has traditionally been indicated by the colour of the body and shoulder of the cylinder (Table 3.1), although the contents must always be confirmed by checking the attached label. However, recent legislation has proposed that all medical gas cylinders should have a white body with coloured shoulders (see Table 3.1). This change will occur gradually, being complete by 2025. In the interim period, to limit errors, the content will be written on the body of all cylinders. All cylinders have a pin-index safety mechanism to prevent the connection of the wrong cylinder to the wrong terminal on the anaesthetic machine.

Oxygen

Piped oxygen is supplied from a liquid oxygen reserve, where it is stored under pressure (7–10 bar, 1000 kPa) at approximately minus 160 °C in a vacuum-insulated

evaporator (VIE), effectively a large thermos flask. Gaseous oxygen is removed from above the liquid or, at times of increased demand, by vaporizing liquid oxygen using heat from the environment. Th gas is warmed to ambient air temperature en route from the VIE to the pipeline system. A reserve bank of cylinders of compressed oxygen is kept adjacent to the VIE in case the main system fails. A smaller cylinder is attached directly to the anaesthetic machine as an emergency reserve. The pressure in a full cylinder of oxygen is 13 700 kPa (137 bar, 2000 psi) and this falls proportionately as the cylinder empties.

Nitrous oxide

Piped nitrous oxide is supplied from several large cylinders joined together to form a bank and attached to a common manifold. There are usually two banks, one running with all cylinders turned on (duty bank) and a reserve. In addition, there is a small emergency supply. Smaller cylinders are attached directly to the anaesthetic machine. At room temperature, nitrous oxide exists as both a liquid and a vapour within the cylinder. While any liquid remains, the pressure within the cylinder remains constant (5400 kPa, 54 bar, 800 psi). When all the liquid has evaporated, the cylinder contains only vapour and as it empties, the pressure falls to zero.

Medical air

This is supplied either by a compressor or in cylinders. A compressor delivers air to a central reservoir, where it is dried and filtered to achieve the desired quality before distribution. Air is supplied to the operating theatre at 400 kPa for anaesthetic use, and at 700 kPa to power medical tools.

Table 3.1 Medical gas cylinder colours.

Gas	Old colour		New colour	
	Body	Shoulder	Body	Shoulder
Oxygen	Black	White	White	White
Nitrous oxide	Blue	Blue	White	Blue
Entonox	Blue	Blue/white	White	Blue/white
Air	Grey	White/black	White	Black/white
Carbon dioxide	Grey	Grey	White	Grey
Helium/oxygen	Brown	Brown/white	White	Brown/white

Vacuum

The final part of the PMGV system is medical vacuum. Two pumps are connected to a system that must be capable of generating a vacuum of at least 50 kPa below atmospheric pressure. This is delivered to the anaesthetic rooms, operating theatres and other appropriate sites. At several stages between the outlets and the pumps, there are drains and bacterial filters to prevent contamination by aspirated fluids.

The anaesthetic machine

The main functions of the anaesthetic machine are to:

- reduce the high-pressure gases from either the pipeline or cylinders to a pressure that is safe for onward delivery to the patient;
- control the flow of gases, allowing a known, accurate and adjustable composition to be delivered into the anaesthetic breathing system.

In addition to these functions, modern anaesthetic machines usually contain integral monitoring equipment and ventilators.

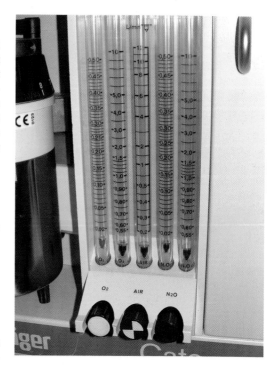

Figure 3.9 Oxygen, air and nitrous oxide flowmeters on an anaesthetic machine.

Reduction of pressure

Cylinders contain gases at very high pressures (see earlier) that can vary depending on the content or temperature of the cylinder. The gas from a cylinder passes through a reducing valve to ensure that a constant flow of gas at 400 kPa is delivered to the flowmeters. As piped gases are already delivered at 400 kPa, no further pressure reduction is required.

Control of flow of gases

Traditionally, on most anaesthetic machines, this has been achieved by the use of flowmeters ('rotameters'; Figure 3.9). A specific, calibrated flowmeter is used for each gas and flow is controlled by a needle valve. A rotating bobbin floats in the gas stream, its upper edge indicating the rate of gas flow.

On modern anaesthetic machines, flowmeters have been replaced with electronic control of gas flow. The anaesthetist simply dials in the required flow and gas composition and this is delivered into the anaesthetic breathing system. The flow of gas is then displayed on a monitor screen either numerically or as a digital representation of a flowmeter.

Anaesthetic machines have several safety features built into the gas delivery system:

- the oxygen and nitrous oxide controls are linked, preventing less than 25% oxygen from being delivered;
- an emergency oxygen 'flush' device can be used to deliver pure oxygen at greater than 40 L/minute into the breathing system;
- an audible alarm to warn of failure of oxygen delivery – this discontinues the nitrous oxide supply and if the patient is breathing spontaneously, air can be entrained;
- a non-return valve to minimize the effects of back-pressure on the function of flowmeters and vaporizers.

Addition of anaesthetic vapours

This is achieved by the use of vaporizers, devices that produce a very accurate concentration of each inhalational anaesthetic drug (Figure 3.10).

- Vaporizers produce a saturated vapour from a reservoir of liquid anaesthetic.

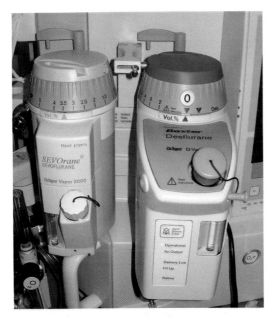

Figure 3.10 Sevoflurane vaporizer (*left*) and desflurane vaporizer (*right*) on an anaesthetic machine. Note the interlock positioned between the coloured dials to prevent simultaneous delivery of both vapours.

- The final concentration of anaesthetic is controlled by varying the proportion of gas passing into the vapour chamber.
- Vaporization of the anaesthetic results in loss of latent heat, causing the remaining anaesthetic liquid to cool and reducing further vaporization. This would result in a fall in the concentration of anaesthetic delivered to the patient. To circumvent this problem, vaporizers incorporate a mechanism to compensate for the fall in temperature.
- Most anaesthetic machines allow more than one vaporizer to be fitted at any time. To prevent accidental delivery of more than one vapour, an 'interlock' is fitted. This is usually a mechanical device that prevents more than one vaporizer being turned on simultaneously.

The resultant mixture of gases and vapour is finally delivered to a common outlet on the anaesthetic machine. From this point, specialized breathing systems are used to transfer the gases and vapours to the patient.

Anaesthetic breathing systems

The mixture of gases and anaesthetic vapour travels from the anaesthetic machine to the patient via an anaesthetic 'circuit' or, more correctly, an anaesthetic breathing system, and finally to the patient's lungs via a facemask, supraglottic airway or tracheal tube. Historically, a number of different breathing systems were used but nowadays these have largely been replaced by circle systems. The details of these systems are beyond the scope of this book but they all have a number of common features, described later. As several patients in succession may breathe through the same system, a low-resistance, disposable bacterial filter is placed at the patient end of the system, and changed between each patient to reduce the risk of cross-infection. Alternatively, a disposable system can be used, which is changed between each patient.

Components of a breathing system

All systems consist of the following.

- *A connection for fresh gas input:* connects to the common gas outlet on the anaesthetic machine.
- *A reservoir bag:* usually of 2 L capacity. This serves several purposes: it allows the patient's peak inspiratory demands (30–40 L/minute) to be met with a lower constant flow from the anaesthetic machine, manual ventilation of the patient if needed, and an indication of ventilation in a spontaneously breathing patient. It also acts as a further safety device, being easily distended at low pressure if obstruction occurs.
- *An adjustable pressure-limiting (APL) valve:* to vent expired gas, helping to eliminate carbon dioxide. During spontaneous ventilation, resistance to opening is minimal so as not to impede expiration. Closing the valve and squeezing the reservoir bag allows the generation of positive pressure within the breathing system and therefore manual ventilation of the patient.

The circle system

Many traditional anaesthetic breathing systems used high flows of gases and vapour to prevent rebreathing of expired gases and hypercapnia. The expired gas was vented to the atmosphere, thereby 'wasting' the unused, exhaled oxygen and anaesthetic vapour it contained. The circle system (Figure 3.11) overcomes this inefficiency by 'recycling' some of the expired gas mixture and as a result, gas flows from the anaesthetic machine can be as low as 0.3–0.5 L/minute.

- The expired gases are passed through a container of soda lime (the absorber), a mixture of calcium, sodium and potassium hydroxide that chemically removes carbon dioxide.

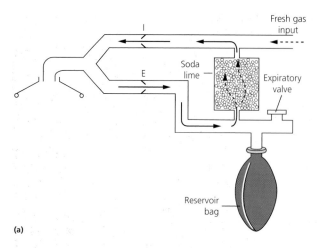

(a)

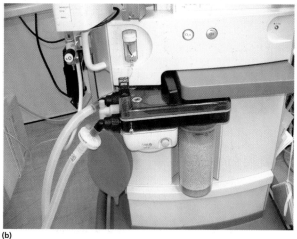

(b)

Figure 3.11 (a) Diagrammatic representation of a circle system (I, inspiratory; E, expiratory valves). (b) Circle system on an anaesthetic machine. Most of the components shown in the diagram are integrated; only the inspiratory and expiratory tubing, the reservoir bag and soda lime container are obvious.

- After the carbon dioxide has been removed, the expired gas has supplementary oxygen and anaesthetic vapour added to maintain the desired concentrations, and the mixture is rebreathed by the patient.
- As the gases pass through the absorber, they are warmed and humidified as a consequence of the reaction that removes carbon dioxide.

There are several points to note when using a circle system.

- The inspired gas is a mixture of expired and fresh gas. Its composition is affected by a number of factors including uptake of anaesthetic by the patient and fresh gas flow. As a result, the concentration of oxygen and anaesthetic vapour within the circle does not correlate with what has been set on the anaesthetic machine or vaporizer. For this reason, the inspired oxygen and anaesthetic vapour concentrations must be monitored to ensure that the patient is not:
  o rendered hypoxic;
  o aware, due to an inadequate concentration of anaesthetic;
  o given an excessive concentration of anaesthetic vapour.
- An indicator is incorporated into the soda lime so that when it is unable to absorb any more carbon dioxide, the granules change colour. One of the commonly used preparations changes from pink to white.
- A standard circle system has an internal volume of 6 L, so after a change in the composition of fresh gas mixture there will be a delay of several minutes before the gas mixture in the circle equilibrates. The lower the fresh gas flow rate, the longer this lag time will be.

Patients can either breathe spontaneously or be ventilated when using the circle system.

Mechanical ventilation

A wide variety of anaesthetic ventilators is available, each of which functions in a slightly different way. The following is an outline of the principles of mechanical ventilation; more details are available in the Further information section at the end of the chapter.

During spontaneous ventilation, negative intrathoracic pressure is generated, causing gas to move into the lungs. This process is reversed during mechanical ventilation. A positive pressure is applied to the anaesthetic gases to overcome airway resistance and elastic recoil of the chest, causing gas flow into the lungs. This technique is usually referred to as intermittent positive pressure ventilation (IPPV). In order to generate the positive pressure, the ventilator requires a source of energy – generally gas pressure or electricity. In both spontaneous and mechanical ventilation, expiration occurs by passive recoil of the lungs and chest wall.

When using a mechanical ventilator, the following can be controlled:

- tidal volume;
- respiratory rate;
- the mode of ventilation, usually a choice between volume and pressure controlled;
- the inspiratory and expiratory times;
- peak inspiratory pressure;
- the use of and magnitude of positive end expiratory pressure (PEEP).

Modes of ventilation

Anaesthetists can select the tidal volume that they want the ventilator to deliver to the patient. This is volume-controlled ventilation. The resulting pressure generated within the airway is dependent on the volume set and the compliance of the patient's respiratory system. The preset volume will be delivered but this may result in high airway pressures and damage to the lungs (barotrauma) if there is poor respiratory compliance. The alternative is to set the maximum airway pressure generated by the ventilator. The pressure set and the patient's respiratory compliance determine the tidal volume. This is called pressure-controlled ventilation (PCV). Whilst its use reduces the risk of barotrauma, it could lead to the delivery of excessive tidal volumes, resulting in volutrauma. A third ventilator mode found on anaesthetic machines is pressure support ventilation (PSV). This is used when the

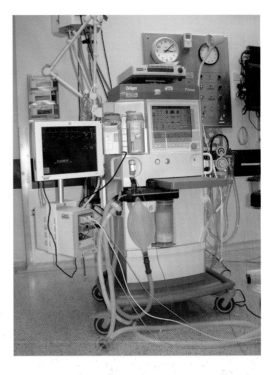

Figure 3.12 Modern integrated anaesthetic machine and monitors.

patient is breathing spontaneously but their own respiratory effort results in inadequate tidal volumes. In this case, the anaesthetist can set the ventilator to detect a spontaneous breath and then provide a little positive pressure to help increase the tidal volume.

In all of these modes, PEEP can be applied to try and prevent the alveolar collapse that occurs when a patient is under general anaesthesia, improve respiratory compliance and improve ventilation/perfusion matching.

The modern anaesthetic machine

Advances in technology have allowed virtually all of the above functions to be integrated into a single unit (Figure 3.12). Electronic controls (Figure 3.13) then allow the anaesthetist to determine:

- spontaneous or controlled ventilation;
- the flow of each gas required;
- the inspired oxygen concentration.

Some machines allow the vapour concentration to be set; on others, the concentration from the vaporizer is set and adjusted to achieve the required end-tidal concentration. All of the above are monitored and

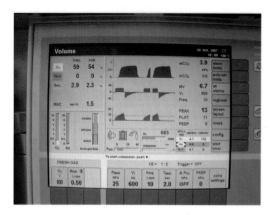

Figure 3.13 Close-up of controls and display of the anaesthetic machine in Figure 3.12.

displayed, and can be set to alarm if they fall outside predetermined limits. In case of power failure, there is a back-up battery supply to maintain key operations and, if this fails, the patient can still be ventilated manually.

Minimizing theatre pollution

Unless special measures are taken, the atmosphere in the operating theatre would become polluted with anaesthetic gases. The breathing systems and mechanical ventilators described vent varying volumes of excess and expired gas into the atmosphere, the patient expires anaesthetic gas during recovery and there are leaks from anaesthetic apparatus. Although no conclusive evidence exists to link prolonged exposure to low concentrations of inhalational anaesthetics with any risks, it would seem sensible to minimize the degree of pollution within the operating theatre environment. This can be achieved in a number of ways:

- use of scavenging systems;
- reducing the flow of gases, for example by use of a circle system;
- avoiding the use of gases, for example by use of total intravenous anaesthesia (TIVA) (see Chapter 5) or regional anaesthesia;
- using air conditioning in the theatre.

Scavenging systems

These collect the gas vented from breathing systems and ventilators and deliver it via a pipeline system to the external atmosphere. The most widely used is an active system in which a small negative pressure is applied to the expiratory valve of the breathing system or ventilator to remove gases to the outside environment. The patient is protected against excessive negative pressure being applied to the lungs by valves with very low opening pressures. The use of such systems does not eliminate the problem of pollution; it merely transfers it from one site to another. Unfortunately, both nitrous oxide and, to a lesser extent, the inhalational anaesthetics are potent destroyers of ozone, thereby adding to the greenhouse effect.

Intravascular cannulas

All patients undergoing anaesthesia need intravenous access in order to administer fluids, blood and drugs. There is a range of different lengths and diameters available and in general the term 'cannula' is used for those less than 7 cm in length and 'catheter' for those more than 7 cm long. The external diameter is quoted in terms of its gauge (G), and also in millimetres, and the maximum flow rate is usually quoted on the packet. The main types of cannula used are as follows.

- *Cannula over needle:* the commonest design, available in sizes ranging from 14 G (2.1 mm) to 24 G (0.7 mm) and colour coded according to size. It consists of a plastic cannula mounted on a metal needle with the bevel protruding. At the other end of the needle is a transparent 'flashback chamber', which can be seen to fill with blood once the needle bevel lies within the vein. All devices have a Luer-Lok™ fitting for attachment to a giving set. Some devices have 'wings' so an adhesive dressing can be used to stick it to the skin and some have a valved injection port for administering drugs. Manufacturers have developed 'safety' versions of their cannulas, which incorporate a way of covering the sharp bevel of the needle once it is removed from the cannula to prevent needle-stick injuries and these are becoming increasingly popular (Figure 3.14).
- *Seldinger type:* these are mainly used for central venous catheterization. Peripheral devices are available and are usually of large diameter for use when large flow rates are needed.

Some patients may require an arterial line for close monitoring of their blood pressure (see later). There are two commonly used devices to achieve this. The first resembles a cannula over needle intravenous cannula except that the valved injection port is removed (to prevent mistaken intra-arterial drug

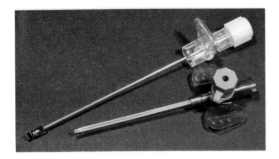

Figure 3.14 Safety cannula. Once the needle is withdrawn from the cannula, the tip is protected to reduce the risk of a needle-stick injury.

injection) and replaced with a flow-switch. The second type of device is a small Seldinger cannula. Both are made of plastic and are parallel sided. In adults, 20 G cannulas are usually used for radial artery cannulation.

Giving sets and fluid warmers

Fluid and blood are administered to the patient from a bag hung on a drip stand through a giving set connected to the Luer-Lok fitting on the intravenous cannula. Different giving sets exist for different purposes; some are designed to be used specifically with certain makes of infusion pumps. In general, giving sets for intravenous fluids have a single drip chamber without a filter and narrower diameter tubing. Giving sets for use with blood and blood products have an additional drip chamber with a mesh filter to filter out any clots and wider diameter tubing.

Intravenous fluids are often at ambient temperature (20 °C), while blood and blood products may be as cold as 4 °C when given, which can lead to significant cooling of the patient; to prevent this, fluids are often warmed as they are being given. This can be achieved by passing the fluid through a section of a giving set with two concentric lumens, where the outer lumen contains a warming fluid, or by passing the fluid past heated plates. Different systems have varying maximum flow rates and varying efficiencies, but the aim is to heat the fluid being infused to as close to body temperature as possible.

Patient warming

Most patients' core temperature falls during anaesthesia as a result of exposure to a cold environment, evaporation of fluids from body cavities, being given cold intravenous fluids and breathing relatively dry, cold anaesthetic gases. This is compounded by the loss of body temperature regulation and inability to shiver when anaesthetized. Hypothermia is associated with delayed recovery and increased postoperative complications and so measures must be taken to try and prevent it. The commonest technique used is forced air warming, a process in which warm air is blown over the surface of the patient that is not exposed for surgery via a perforated blanket (single patient use). Alternative methods are to lie the patient on a mattress heated either electrically or by perfusion with warm water.

Cell savers

These machines are used to reduce the need for allogenic blood transfusion where significant bleeding is expected, for example aortic aneurysm surgery, cardiac surgery and major orthopaedic surgery. The machine incorporates a suction unit that the surgeon uses to collect the patient's blood from the surgical field. This collected blood is then mixed with heparinized saline or anticoagulant citrate dextrose solution A (ACD-A) to prevent it clotting, passed though a filter to remove fat and other debris and then centrifuged to remove all other blood cells and plasma, leaving a concentrate of red cells. These are then resuspended in solution ready for transfusion back to the patient.

Ultrasound

This uses very high-frequency sound waves emitted from a probe and reflected back from body tissues to detect changes in tissue density. A computer then interprets the reflected waves and constructs an image that can be displayed on a screen to visualize a patient's anatomy. Recently there has been increasing use of ultrasound by anaesthetists to guide needle placement during procedures such as central venous catheter insertion or peripheral nerve blocks. The aim is that keeping the needle tip under constant vision during the procedure will reduce the chance of complications and increase effectiveness of nerve blocks by better placement of local anaesthetic. Ultrasound is also increasingly being used for diagnostic purposes in trauma and in emergency life support, for example focused assessment with sonography in trauma (FAST scanning) and focused echocardiography in emergency life support (FEEL). In the ITU, ultrasound has become an invaluable diagnostic and monitoring tool, for example to look for pleural and pericardial effusions and estimate cardiac function (filling, contractility, valve function).

Syringe pumps

Simple syringe pumps can be programmed to deliver an infusion of a drug at a certain rate (mL/hour), and stop after a certain volume. They are accurate over a wide range of infusion rates, usually 0.1 mL/hour to 1000 mL/hour or greater. They also incorporate alarms, for example if there is a high resistance to infusion. More sophisticated syringe pumps are available that use complicated mathematical models to predict the plasma and central nervous system (CNS) concentrations of drugs being infused, for example propofol and remifentanil. The anaesthetist enters patient details such as sex, body mass index (BMI), age and the target concentration, and the syringe pump will calculate and adjust the necessary infusion rate. This is called target-controlled infusion (TCI). It allows for delivery of appropriate concentrations of drugs, enabling accurate titration of effect such that patients can undergo conscious sedation or TIVA [3.4].

Measurement and monitoring

Measurement and monitoring are closely linked but are not synonymous. A measuring instrument becomes a monitor if it is capable of delivering a warning when the variable being measured falls outside preset limits. During anaesthesia, both the patient and the equipment being used are monitored.

Monitoring the patient

Monitoring of the electrocardiogram (ECG), blood pressure (non-invasive), pulse oximetry, capnometry, and oxygen and vapour concentrations is now regarded as essential for the safe conduct of anaesthesia. Various other parameters may also be monitored depending on the patient and the operation [3.5].

ECG

This is easily applied and gives information on heart rate and rhythm, and may indicate the presence of ischaemia and acute disturbances of certain electrolytes (for example, potassium and calcium). It can be monitored using three leads – one applied to the right shoulder (red), another to the left shoulder (yellow) and a third to the left lower chest (green), which will give a tracing equivalent to standard lead II of the 12-lead ECG. Many ECG monitors now use five electrodes placed on the anterior chest to allow all the standard leads and V5 to be displayed. The ECG alone gives no information on the adequacy of the cardiac output and it must be remembered that it is possible to have a virtually normal ECG with minimal cardiac output.

Non-invasive blood pressure

This is the commonest method of monitoring the patient's blood pressure during anaesthesia and surgery. Auscultation of the Korotkoff sounds is difficult in the operating theatre, so automated devices are widely used. An electrical pump inflates a cuff, commonly placed around the arm over the brachial artery. The cuff then undergoes controlled deflation. A microprocessor-controlled pressure transducer detects variations in cuff pressure resulting from transmitted arterial pulsations. Initial pulsations represent systolic blood pressure and peak amplitude of the pulsations equates to mean arterial pressure. Diastolic is then calculated using an algorithm.

The pneumatic cuff must have a width that is **40% of the arm circumference** and the internal inflatable bladder should encircle at least half the arm. If the cuff is too small, the blood pressure will be overestimated, and if it is too large it will be underestimated. The frequency of blood pressure estimation can be set, and the monitor can be set to alarm if the recorded blood pressure falls outside predetermined limits. Such devices cannot measure pressure continually, and become increasingly inaccurate at extremes of pressure and in patients with an arrhythmia.

Pulse oximeter

A probe, containing a light-emitting diode (LED) and a photodetector, is applied across the tip of a digit or earlobe. The LED emits light, alternating between two different wavelengths in the visible and infrared regions of the electromagnetic spectrum. These are transmitted through the tissues and absorbed to different degrees by the tissues, oxyhaemoglobin and deoxyhaemoglobin. The intensity of light reaching the photodetector is converted to an electrical signal. Absorption by the tissues and venous blood is constant but absorption by arterial blood varies with the cardiac cycle, which allows determination of the peripheral arterial oxygen saturation (SpO_2), as both a waveform and a digital reading. This waveform can also be interpreted to give a reading of heart rate.

Pulse oximeters are accurate to ±2% with $SpO_2 > 90\%$. Alarms can be set for levels of saturation and heart rate. Therefore, the pulse oximeter gives information about both the circulatory and respiratory systems and has the advantages of:

- providing continuous monitoring of oxygenation at tissue level;
- being unaffected by skin pigmentation;
- portability (mains or battery powered);
- being non-invasive.

Despite this, there are a number of important limitations with this device.

- There could be a failure to appreciate the severity of hypoxia. Because of the shape of the haemoglobin dissociation curve, a saturation of 90% equates to a PaO_2 of 8 kPa (60 mmHg).
- The pulse oximeter is not an indicator of the adequacy of alveolar ventilation as hypoventilation can be compensated for by increasing the inspired oxygen concentration to maintain oxygen saturation.
- It is unreliable when there is severe vasoconstriction due to the reduced pulsatile component of the signal.
- It is unreliable with certain haemoglobins:
  - carboxyhaemoglobin: results in overestimation of SaO_2;
  - methaemoglobinaemia: at an $SaO_2 > 85\%$ results in underestimation of the saturation.
- It progressively underreads the saturation as the haemoglobin falls (but it is not affected by polycythaemia).
- It is affected by extraneous light.
- It is unreliable when there is excessive movement of the patient.

In many modern anaesthetic systems, the above monitors are integrated and displayed on a single screen (Figure 3.15).

Capnometry

The capnometer (often referred to as a capnograph) works on the principle that carbon dioxide (CO_2) absorbs infrared light in proportion to its concentration. In a healthy person, the CO_2 concentration in air at the end of expiration (end-tidal CO_2, $PetCO_2$) correlates well with the partial pressure in arterial blood ($PaCO_2$), the former being lower,

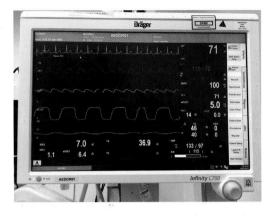

Figure 3.15 Integrated monitor displaying ECG and heart rate, invasive blood pressure (arterial waveform), pulse oximeter waveform, end-tidal carbon dioxide concentration and waveform, inspired and expired oxygen and desflurane concentrations, saturation and temperature.

by 5 mmHg or 0.7 kPa. Continual analysis of CO_2 during ventilation will produce a waveform, referred to as waveform capnography, and is primarily used as an indicator of the adequacy of ventilation; $PaCO_2$ is inversely proportional to alveolar ventilation. In patients with a low cardiac output (for example, hypovolaemia, pulmonary embolus), the gap between arterial and end-tidal carbon dioxide increases (end-tidal falls), mainly due to the development of increased areas of ventilation/perfusion mismatch. The gap also increases in patients with chest disease due to poor mixing of respiratory gases. Care must be taken in interpreting end-tidal CO_2 concentrations in these circumstances [3.6]. Modern capnographs have alarms for when the end-tidal carbon dioxide is outside preset limits. Other uses of waveform capnography are given in Table 3.2.

Vapour concentration analysis

Whenever a volatile anaesthetic is given, the concentration in the inspired gas mixture should be monitored. This is usually achieved using infrared absorption, similar to carbon dioxide. Each volatile anaesthetic drug will absorb optimally at only one wavelength, and the degree of absorption is dependent on the volatile's concentration. A single device producing the correct wavelengths can be calibrated for all of the commonly used inhalational anaesthetics.

Table 3.2 Uses of waveform capnography.

- An indicator of the degree of alveolar ventilation to:
  - ensure normocapnia during mechanical ventilation
  - control the level of hypocapnia in neurosurgery
  - avoid hypocapnia where the cerebral circulation is impaired, e.g. in the elderly
- As a disconnection indicator (the reading suddenly falls to zero)
- To indicate that the tracheal tube is in the trachea (CO_2 in expired gas)
- As an indicator of the degree of rebreathing (presence of CO_2 in inspired gas)
- As an indicator of cardiac output. If cardiac output falls and ventilation is maintained, then end-tidal CO_2 falls as CO_2 is not delivered to the lungs, e.g.:
  - hypovolaemia
  - cardiac arrest, where it can be used to indicate effectiveness of external cardiac compression, and return of spontaneous circulation
  - massive pulmonary embolus
- It may be the first clue to the development of malignant hyperpyrexia

Peripheral nerve stimulator

This is used to assess neuromuscular blockade after giving neuromuscular blocking drugs, for example at the end of surgery, to see if the neuromuscular block has reduced sufficiently to allow for reversal. A peripheral nerve supplying a discrete muscle group is stimulated transcutaneously with a current of 50 mA. The resulting contractions are observed or measured. One arrangement is to stimulate the ulnar nerve at the wrist whilst monitoring the contractions (twitch) of the adductor pollicis. Although most often done by looking at or feeling the response, measuring either the force of contraction or the compound action potential is more objective. Sequences of stimulation used include:

- four stimuli each of 0.2 millisecond duration, at 2 Hz for 1.5 seconds, referred to as a 'train-of-four' (TOF);
- one stimulus at 50 Hz of 5 seconds duration – that is, a tetanic stimulus;
- two groups of three tetanic bursts at 50 Hz, 750 milliseconds apart, called double-burst stimulation (DBS).

During non-depolarizing neuromuscular blockade, there is a progressive decremental response to all the sequences, termed 'fade'. In the TOF, the ratio of the amplitude of the fourth twitch (T4) to the first twitch (T1) is used as an index of the degree of neuromuscular blockade. The absence of any response is seen either with profound neuromuscular block, for example shortly after a drug has been given, or is the result of failure to deliver a stimulus. During depolarizing blockade, the response to all sequences of stimulation is reduced but consistent; that is, there is no fade.

Temperature

During anaesthesia, the patient's temperature should be monitored continually in accordance with recent NICE guidelines [3.7]. The most commonly used device is a thermistor, a semiconductor that varies in resistance according to its temperature. This can be placed in the oesophagus (cardiac temperature) or nasopharynx (brain temperature). The rectum can be used but, apart from being unpleasant, faeces may insulate the thermistor, leading to inaccuracies. Urinary catheters are available with thermistors built in to the tip, which monitors temperature in the bladder. An infrared tympanic membrane thermometer can be used intermittently, but the external auditory canal must be clear. Although temperature is normally measured to help identify and prevent hypothermia, a sudden unexpected rise in a patient's temperature may be the first warning of the development of malignant hyperpyrexia (see Chapter 4).

Invasive or direct blood pressure

This is the most accurate method for measuring and monitoring blood pressure and is generally reserved for use in complex, prolonged surgery or sick patients. A cannula is inserted into a peripheral artery and connected via a fluid-filled tube to a transducer that converts the pulsatile pressure signal into an electrical signal. This is then amplified and displayed as both the arterial waveform and systolic, diastolic and mean arterial blood pressures (see Figure 3.15).

Central venous pressure (CVP)

This is measured by inserting a catheter via a central vein (central venous catheter, CVC), usually the internal jugular or subclavian, so that its tip lies at the junction of the superior vena cava and right atrium. It is then connected as described above to display a waveform and pressure.

Table 3.3 Factors affecting the central venous pressure.

- The zero reference point
- Patient posture
- Fluid status
- Heart failure
- Raised intrathoracic pressure:
  - mechanical ventilation
  - coughing
  - straining
- Pulmonary embolism
- Pulmonary hypertension
- Tricuspid valve disease
- Pericardial effusion, tamponade
- Superior vena cava obstruction

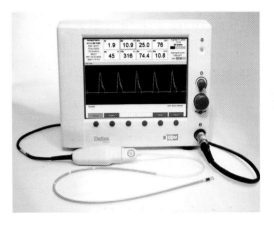

Figure 3.16 Transoesophageal Doppler monitor and oesophageal probe. Reproduced with permission of Deltex Medical.

Although absolute values of the CVP can be measured, its trend is usually more informative. Often a 'fluid challenge' is used in the face of a low CVP. The CVP is measured, a rapid infusion of fluid is given and the change in CVP noted. In the hypovolaemic patient, the CVP increases briefly and then falls back to around the previous value, whereas in the euvolaemic patient the CVP will show a greater and more sustained rise. Overtransfusion will be seen as a high, sustained CVP.

Central venous pressure is usually monitored during operations in which there is the potential for major fluid shifts or blood loss, or in those patients in whom even small fluid shifts may be detrimental, for example heart failure. It is affected by a variety of other factors apart from fluid balance (Table 3.3), in particular cardiac function and positive pressure ventilation. Hypotension in the presence of an elevated CVP (absolute or in response to a fluid challenge) may indicate heart failure. However, most clinicians would now accept that in these circumstances monitoring left ventricular function with either transoesophageal Doppler or one of the pulse analysis cardiac output monitoring devices is preferable.

Oesophageal Doppler cardiac output monitoring

Insertion of an oesophageal Doppler probe is relatively non-invasive, the ultrasound emitter-sensor being passed into the oesophagus to lie just in front of the descending aorta, in a technique similar to that of

inserting a nasogastric tube (Figure 3.16). The underlying principle behind it is that flow through a cylinder (aorta) can be calculated from its cross-sectional area and the velocity of the fluid (measured using Doppler shift). Previous devices calculated the blood flow in the descending aorta and applied correction factors for upper body blood flow to calculate total cardiac output. Current devices (e.g. CardioQODM™) use a nomogram incorporating age, weight and height and cardiac output values measured by thermodilution using a pulmonary artery catheter to convert measured descending aortic blood flow velocity into total cardiac output for each patient. This eliminates the need to make allowances for blood flow to the upper body, which can be a significant source of error. Monitoring is continuous, acute changes in cardiac output can be detected and because flow is measured in the aorta, its accuracy is not affected by changes in peripheral resistance. Optimal results require alignment of the oesophageal probe with the axial blood flow, which may mean minor adjustments of the probe position. The oesophageal Doppler is a useful tool, particularly in following trends in cardiac output following fluid challenges (Figure 3.17), and is now well established in major abdominal surgery.

Pulse analysis cardiac output monitoring

There are three systems currently available.

- *PiCCO®:* pulse contour continuous cardiac output monitoring. This requires a CVC and specialized arterial catheter placed in a large artery, such as

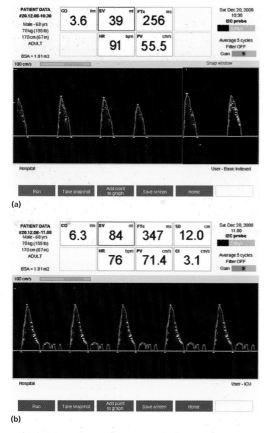

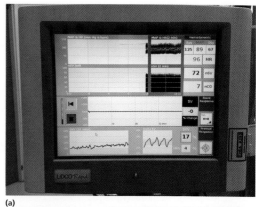

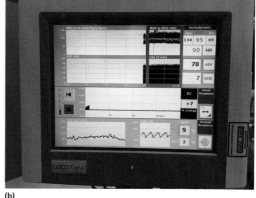

Figure 3.17 (a) Narrow waveform typical of hypovolaemia. Note: Cardiac output (CO) 3.6 L/minute, stroke volume (SV) 39 mL, heart rate (HR) 91/minute. (b) Broadening of the waveform after giving the patient an IV fluid challenge. Note improvement in haemodynamics: CO 6.3 L/minute, SV 84 mL, HR 76/minute. Reproduced with permission of Deltex Medical.

Figure 3.18 (a) Pulse contour (LIthium Dilution Cardiac Output (LiDCO)) monitor. Note: BP 125/67 mmHg, MAP 89 mmHg, HR 96/minute, stroke volume (nSV) 72 mL, stroke volume variation (SVV) 17%. (b) After a fluid challenge, note improvement in haemodynamics: BP 134/69 mmHg, mean arterial pressure (MAP) 95 mmHg, HR 90/minute, nSV 78 mL, SVV 9%.

the femoral artery. Calibration is performed by injecting a fixed volume of cold saline via the CVC and detecting the resulting drop in blood temperature via the arterial catheter to calculate cardiac output. Following this, the arterial waveform is continually analysed and cardiac output calculated by reference to the calibration reading.
- *LiDCO®:* lithium dilution continuous cardiac output. This requires peripheral IV and arterial cannulas. Calibration is performed by injecting a known amount of lithium chloride through the IV cannula. The change in blood lithium concentration is measured by drawing blood from

the arterial cannula past a lithium sensor and cardiac output is calculated from this. Following this, the arterial pulse pressure is continuously monitored and by reference to the calibration readings, cardiac output is derived from an algorithm that relates pulse pressure to blood flow (Figure 3.18).

Both of the above systems require regular recalibration.

- *Flotrac®:* this is an uncalibrated system and only requires an arterial cannula to function. This is attached to a specialized transducer and monitor that allow detailed analysis of the arterial waveform that in turn calculates stroke volume. As pulse rate is measured, cardiac output can be calculated. The only other information required is the patient's age, sex and weight to allow compliance to be estimated.

All three systems require high-quality arterial wave-forms, with no damping, to allow correct evaluation of cardiac output.

Bispectral index (BIS)

This is a method for monitoring the depth of anaesthesia (Figure 3.19). General anaesthesia alters the electroencephalogram (EEG) with a general reduction in activity with increasing depth of anaesthesia. Bispectral index records the complex and difficult to interpret raw EEG data and processes it using proprietary software to produce a number between 0 (no cortical electrical activity) and 100 (fully awake), which can be used to indicate the risk of recall or awareness. When used, most operators would accept a numerical value between 40 and 60 as appropriate for general anaesthesia. Situations where BIS may be useful include when it is not possible to monitor inspired and expired volatile anaesthetic concentrations, for example during cardiopulmonary bypass, when using TIVA and relying on predicted plasma concentrations, avoidance of excessive anaesthesia in haemodynamically unstable patients, and in those with a previous episode of awareness under general anaesthesia.

Blood loss

Strictly speaking, this is measured rather than monitored. Simple estimates of blood loss during surgery are easily performed. Swabs can be weighed, dry and wet, the increase in weight giving an indication of the amount of blood they have absorbed. The volume of blood in the suction apparatus can be measured, with allowance for irrigation fluids. Such methods are only estimates, as blood may remain in body cavities, be spilt on the floor and absorbed by drapes and gowns. In paediatric practice, where small volumes of blood loss are relatively more important, all absorbent materials are washed to remove the blood and the resultant solvent analysed by colorimetry to estimate blood loss.

Many other physiological parameters can be, and are, measured during anaesthesia when appropriate. Some examples are clotting profiles and haemoglobin concentration in patients receiving a transfusion of a large volume of stored blood; blood glucose in diabetic patients; and arterial blood gas and acid–base

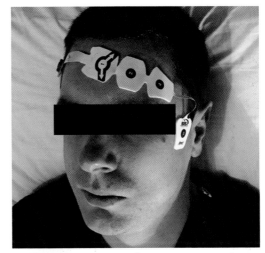

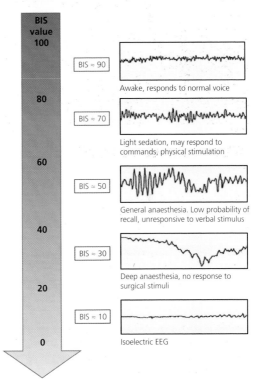

Figure 3.19 BIS device and representative features for given BIS values.

analysis during the cardiopulmonary bypass phase of cardiac surgery.

It is essential to recognize that the above standards apply not only to those patients undergoing general anaesthesia, but also those receiving sedation, local or regional anaesthesia and during transfer.

Finally, one should never rely solely on monitors – regular observation and examination of the patient and clinical judgement are essential to avoid acting on false information.

Monitoring the equipment

With the increasing reliance on complex equipment to deliver anaesthesia, the AAGBI recommends that there should be continuous monitoring of the oxygen supply and correct functioning of the breathing system.

Oxygen supply

All anaesthetic machines are fitted with a device warning of oxygen supply failure. Continuous monitoring of the oxygen concentration in the inspired gas mixture is considered essential. This is usually achieved using a fuel cell oxygen analyser that produces a current proportional to the oxygen concentration, displayed as a numeric value of oxygen concentration. **It must be remembered that the inspired oxygen concentration does not guarantee adequate arterial oxygen saturation** as it may be insufficient to compensate for the effects of hypoventilation and ventilation/perfusion mismatch (see Chapter 8).

Breathing systems

Irrespective of whether the patient is breathing spontaneously or being ventilated, capnometry will alert the anaesthetist to most of the common problems, for example disconnection (loss of reading), exhaustion of the CO_2 absorber (failure of the reading to fall to zero during inspiration), inadequate gas flow (increased end-tidal CO_2 although hypoxia is a greater risk), hyper/hypoventilation (decreased/increased end-tidal CO_2, respectively). In addition, when a patient is mechanically ventilated, airway pressures must be monitored to avoid excessive pressures being generated within the lungs. Airway pressure monitoring can also be used as a secondary indicator of inadequate ventilation in ventilated patients; high pressures may be the result of obstruction (for example, blocked tracheal tube, bronchospasm), and loss of pressure may be the result of a disconnection. The latter function may be specifically used as a 'disconnection alarm'.

FURTHER INFORMATION

Aitkenhead AR, Moppett IK, Thompson JP (eds). *Smith and Aitkenhead's Textbook of Anaesthesia*, 6th edn. Edinburgh: Churchill Livingstone, 2013.

Al-Shaikh B, Stacey S. *Essentials of anaesthetic equipment*, 4th edn. Edinburgh: Churchill Livingstone Elsevier, 2013.

Cook T, Howes B. Supraglottic airway devices: recent advances. *Continuing Education in Anaesthesia, Critical Care and Pain* 2011; **11**(2): 56–61.

McGuire BE, Younger RA. Rigid indirect laryngoscopy and optical stylets. *Continuing Education in Anaesthesia, Critical Care and Pain* 2010; **10**(5): 148–151.

Patel B, Frerk C. Large bore cricothyroidotomy devices. *Continuing Education in Anaesthesia, Critical Care and Pain* 2008; **8**(5): 157–160.

Yentis SM, Hirsch NP, Ip J. *Anaesthesia and Intensive Care A to Z: An Encyclopaedia of Principles and Practice*, 5th edn. Edinburgh: Churchill Livingstone, 2013.

[3.1] www.mhra.gov.uk/
Medicines and Healthcare products Regulatory Agency (UK) ensures that medicines, healthcare products and medical equipment meet appropriate standards of safety, quality, performance and effectiveness, and are used safely. Report adverse events to this agency in the UK.

[3.2] www.frca.co.uk/
Anaesthesia UK. A popular web site for trainees in anaesthesia.

[3.3] www.theairwaysite.com/pages/page_content/airway_equipment.aspx
This site is aimed at emergency physicians and orientated to American practice. It does, however, contain some useful information about airway equipment.

[3.4] www.siva.ac.uk
Web site of the Society for Intravenous Anaesthesia.

[3.5] https://www.aagbi.org/sites/default/files/standardsofmonitoring07.pdf
AAGBI Recommendations for Standards of Monitoring during Anaesthesia and Recovery.

[3.6] www.capnography.com/index.html
This is an excellent site if you want to know more about capnography. Very detailed, so be warned.

[3.7] https://www.nice.org.uk/guidance/cg65
NICE guidance on the prevention and management of hypothermia in adults undergoing surgery.

4

Drugs and fluids used during anaesthesia

Learning objectives

After reading this chapter you should understand the principles of:

☐ The basic pharmacology of the drugs used for induction and maintenance of anaesthesia and neuromuscular blockade

☐ The basic pharmacology of the analgesic drugs and antiemetics

☐ The basic pharmacology of local anaesthetic drugs and their regulation

☐ The different types of fluids used in the perioperative period, including crystalloids, colloids, blood and its components

☐ The indications for and limitations of the different fluids available

Apply this knowledge when practising the following skills:

☐ Calculating the maximum safe dose of drugs for a given patient and procedure

☐ Under supervision, preparing the correct doses of drugs for induction of anaesthesia

☐ Under supervision, preparing the correct doses of drugs for neuromuscular blockade

---

Anaesthetists have to be familiar with a wide range of drugs, those directly associated with anaesthesia, and also any medications taken by a patient that may impact upon anaesthesia [2.2]. Unlike in most other branches of medicine, drugs associated with anaesthesia are almost always given parenterally, either intravenously or via inhalation, usually produce rapid and profound physiological changes, and may have serious undesirable actions in addition to their intended effects. As well as drugs, many patients will also require intravenous fluids, blood and blood products perioperatively. All drugs given in the UK are regulated by the Medicines and Healthcare products Regulatory Agency (MHRA) [3.1].

Premedication

This refers to any drugs given in the period before induction of anaesthesia, in addition to those normally taken by the patient. Some drugs are given with specific intentions.

Modification of pH and volume of gastric contents

Patients are starved preoperatively to reduce the risk of regurgitation and aspiration of gastric acid at the induction of anaesthesia (see later). However,

Clinical Anaesthesia: Lecture Notes, Fifth Edition. Matthew Gwinnutt and Carl Gwinnutt.
© 2017 John Wiley & Sons, Ltd. Published 2017 by John Wiley & Sons, Ltd.
Companion website: www.lecturenoteseries.com/anaesthesia

certain high-risk groups may be given specific therapy to try to increase the pH and reduce the volume of gastric contents:

- women who are pregnant, particularly in the later stages of pregnancy;
- patients who require emergency surgery;
- patients with a hiatus hernia, who are at an increased risk of regurgitation;
- patients who are morbidly obese.

A variety of drug combinations is used to try and increase the pH and reduce the volume of gastric contents:

- *ranitidine (H1 antagonist)*: 150 mg orally 12 hours and 2 hours preoperatively;
- *omeprazole (proton pump inhibitor)*: 40 mg 3–4 hours preoperatively;
- *metoclopramide*: 10 mg orally preoperatively – it increases both gastric emptying and lower oesophageal sphincter tone and is often given in conjunction with ranitidine;
- *oral sodium citrate (0.3 M)*: 30 mL orally to chemically neutralize residual acid; it is most commonly used immediately before induction of anaesthesia for caesarean section.

If a naso- or orogastric tube is in place, this can be used to aspirate gastric contents.

Analgesia

There has been interest in giving preoperative analgesia to patients who are not in pain prior to surgery, known as 'pre-emptive analgesia'. It is known that tissue damage during surgery leads to an increased sensitivity or upregulation of pain conduction pathways in the peripheral and central nervous systems, making postoperative pain more severe and possibly leading to chronic pain problems. The theory is that giving analgesia before the surgical tissue damage will stop the sensitization, resulting in reduced postoperative pain, which is easier to treat, and preventing chronic pain. So far this approach has not shown a proven benefit.

Patients are sometimes also given oral analgesia (paracetamol or non-steroidal anti-inflammatory drugs (NSAIDs)) prior to short day-case procedures, for example knee arthroscopy and cytoscopy, in order for it to be maximally effective by the end of the operation.

Antiemetics

These drugs are often given as a premed to try and reduce the incidence of postoperative nausea and vomiting (PONV). However, there is increasing evidence that they are more effective if given during or at the end of anaesthesia (see later).

Miscellaneous

A variety of other drugs is commonly given prophylactically before anaesthesia and surgery:

- *steroids*: to patients on long-term treatment, or who have received them within the past 3 months;
- *antibiotics*: to patients with prosthetic or diseased heart valves or undergoing joint replacement or bowel surgery;
- *anticoagulants*: as prophylaxis against deep venous thrombosis;
- *transdermal glyceryl trinitrate (GTN)*: as patches for patients with ischaemic heart disease to reduce the risk of coronary ischaemia;
- *eutectic mixture of local anaesthetics (EMLA)*: a local anaesthetic cream applied topically to reduce the pain of inserting an intravenous (IV) cannula.

The majority of the patient's own regular medications should be taken as normal, unless instructed otherwise by the anaesthetist.

Intravenous anaesthetic drugs

This group of drugs is most commonly used to induce anaesthesia. After IV injection, these drugs are carried in the bloodstream into the cerebral circulation. They are very lipid soluble and quickly cross the blood–brain barrier, resulting in loss of consciousness. Following a single bolus dose, the drug undergoes redistribution to other tissues (initially the muscles and then fat), the plasma and brain concentrations fall and the patient recovers consciousness. Therefore, these drugs have a rapid onset, short duration of action and rapid recovery. Despite this, complete elimination from all tissues of some drugs, usually by hepatic metabolism, takes much longer and repeated doses may lead to accumulation and delayed recovery. This is seen typically with thiopental, and the only exception to this is propofol (see later). All drugs used for induction cause depression of the cardiovascular and respiratory systems and the dose required to induce anaesthesia is significantly reduced in those patients who are elderly, frail, hypovolaemic or have compromise of their cardiovascular system. A synopsis of the drugs commonly used is given in Table 4.1.

Table 4.1 Intravenous drugs used for the induction of anaesthesia and their effects.

Drug CNS	Induction dose (mg/kg)	Speed of induction (seconds)	Duration of action (minutes)	Effects on CVS	Effects on RS	Effects on CNS	Other side-effects	Comments
Propofol	1.5–2.5	30–45	4–7	Hypotension, worse if hypovolaemic or cardiac disease	Apnoea up to 60s, depression of ventilation	Decreases CBF and ICP	Pain on injection, involuntary movement, hiccoughs	Non-cumulative, repeated injections or infusion used to maintain anaesthesia (see TIVA)
Thiopental	2–6	20–30	9–10	Dose-dependent hypotension, worse if hypovolaemic or cardiac disease	Apnoea, depression of ventilation	Decreases CBF and ICP, anticonvulsant	Rare but severe adverse reactions	Patients may 'taste' garlic or onions! Cumulative, delayed recovery after repeat doses
Ketamine	1–2	50–70	10–12	Minimal in fit patients, better tolerated if cardiovascular compromise	Minimal depression of ventilation, laryngeal reflexes better preserved, bronchodilation	CBF maintained, profound analgesia	Vivid hallucinations	Subanaesthetic doses cause analgesia, can be used as sole anaesthetic drug in adverse circumstances, e.g. prehospital
Midazolam	0.1–0.3	40–70	10–15	Dose-dependent hypotension, worse if hypovolaemic or cardiac disease	Depression of ventilation, worse in elderly	Mildly anticonvulsant		Causes amnesia

CBF, cerebral blood flow; CNS, central nervous system; CVS, cardiovascular system; ICP, intracranial pressure; RS, respiratory system; TIVA, total intravenous anaesthesia.

Inhaled anaesthetic drugs

Although these drugs can be used to induce anaesthesia, they are most commonly used to maintain anaesthesia. Apart from nitrous oxide (N_2O), they are halogenated hydrocarbons. They all have relatively low boiling points, evaporate easily at ambient temperature and hence are often referred to as vapours. A controlled amount of the vapour that is produced is added to the fresh gas flow (oxygen and air or nitrous oxide) and breathed by the patient. Once in the lungs, the vapour diffuses into the pulmonary capillary blood and is distributed via the systemic circulation to the brain and other tissues. The depth of anaesthesia produced is directly related to the partial pressure that the vapour exerts in the brain, and this is closely related to the partial pressure in the alveoli. The rate at which the alveolar partial pressure can be changed determines the rate of change in the brain and hence the speed of induction, change in depth and recovery from anaesthesia. Even the most rapid induction using these drugs takes several minutes to achieve the same depth of anaesthesia that is achieved within seconds of giving an IV anaesthetic drug. The inspired concentration of all of these compounds is expressed as the percentage by volume. All the inhalational anaesthetics cause dose-dependent depression of the cardiovascular and respiratory systems. A synopsis of the currently used drugs used is given in Table 4.2.

There are two concepts that will help in understanding the use of inhalational anaesthetics: solubility and minimum alveolar concentration (MAC).

Solubility

The rate of change of depth of anaesthesia is determined by how quickly the partial pressure of anaesthetic can be altered in alveoli, and hence the brain. One of the main factors governing alveolar partial pressure for any given inhalational anaesthetic is its solubility in blood. One that is relatively **soluble** in blood (for example, isoflurane) will dissolve readily in the plasma and exert a low partial pressure. Consequently, a relatively large amount of the anaesthetic has to diffuse from the alveoli before the partial pressure in the blood and the brain begins to rise. Conversely, if an agent is **insoluble** in blood (for example, desflurane), a smaller amount will exert a higher blood and brain partial pressure. Therefore, an increase in depth of anaesthesia can be achieved more quickly. Reducing the depth or recovery from anaesthesia follows similar principles in reverse; a greater amount of a soluble agent will have to be excreted for the brain, blood and alveolar partial pressure to fall, which takes proportionately longer.

Other factors that determine the speed at which the alveolar concentration rises include the following.

- *A high inspired concentration.* This is of limited clinical use due to the pungency of the vapour.
- *Alveolar ventilation.* This is most pronounced for drugs with a high solubility. As large amounts are

Table 4.2 Inhalational anaesthetic drugs and their effects.

Compound	MAC in oxygen/air	Solubility	Effect on CVS	Effect on RS	Effect on CNS	Comments
Sevoflurane	2.2%	Low; rapid changes of depth	↓ BP, vasodilatation	Depresses ventilation	Minimal effect on CBF at clinical concentration	Popular for inhalation induction
Desflurane	6.0%	Low; rapid changes of depth	↓ BP, ↑ HR	Depresses ventilation	Minimal effect on CBF at clinical concentration	Pungent, boils at 23 °C
Isoflurane	1.3%	Medium	↓ BP, ↑ HR, vasodilatation	Depresses ventilation	Slight ↑ CBF and ICP	Pungency limits use for induction

BP, blood pressure; CBF, cerebral blood flow; CNS, central nervous system; CVS, cardiovascular system; ECG, electroencephalograph; HR, heart rate; ICP, intracranial pressure; MAC, minimum alveolar concentration; RS, respiratory system.

removed from the alveoli, increasing ventilation ensures more rapid replacement.

- *Cardiac output*: if high, this results in a greater pulmonary blood flow and increasing uptake, thereby lowering the alveolar partial pressure. If low, the converse occurs and the alveolar concentration rises more rapidly.

Minimum alveolar concentration

To compare the potencies and side-effects of the inhalational anaesthetics, the concept of minimum alveolar concentration (MAC) is used. Minimum alveolar concentration is the concentration required to prevent movement following a surgical stimulus in 50% of subjects. At 1 MAC, or multiples thereof, the anaesthetic effect of different drugs will be the same and a comparison of the side-effects can be made. Compounds with a low potency (such as desflurane) will have a high MAC; those with a higher potency (such as isoflurane) will have a lower MAC.

The effects of inhalational anaesthetics are additive, therefore two values for MAC are often quoted – the value in oxygen (see Table 4.2) and the value when given with a stated percentage of nitrous oxide (which has its own MAC), which will clearly be less. The value of MAC is also affected by a number of other patient factors (Table 4.3).

Table 4.3 Factors affecting the minimum alveolar concentration (MAC) of inhalational anaesthetic drugs.

Increasing MAC	Decreasing MAC
• Infants, children	• Neonates, elderly
• Hyperthermia	• Hypothermia
• Hyperthyroidism	• Hypothyroidism
• Hypernatraemia	• Hyponatraemia
• Chronic alcohol intake	• Acute alcohol intake
• Chronic opioid use	• Acute intake of opioids, benzodiazepines, TCAs, clonidine
• Increased catecholamines	• Lithium, magnesium
	• Pregnancy
	• Anaemia

TCAs, tricyclic antidepressants.

Nitrous oxide

Nitrous oxide (N_2O) is a colourless, sweet-smelling, non-irritant vapour with moderate analgesic properties but low anaesthetic potency (MAC 105%). The maximum safe inspired concentration that can be given without the risk of causing hypoxia is approximately 70%, therefore unconsciousness or anaesthesia sufficient to allow surgery is rarely achieved. Consequently, it is usually given in conjunction with one of the other vapours. Nitrous oxide is available in cylinders premixed with oxygen as a 50:50 mixture called Entonox, which is used as an analgesic in obstetrics and by the emergency services.

Systemic effects of nitrous oxide

- Cardiovascular depression, worse in patients with pre-existing cardiac disease.
- Slight increase in the respiratory rate and a decrease in the tidal volume. It decreases the ventilatory response to hypercapnia and hypoxia.
- Cerebral vasodilatation, increasing intracranial pressure (ICP).
- Diffuses into air-filled cavities more rapidly than nitrogen can escape, causing either a rise in pressure (for example, in the middle ear) or an increase in volume (for example, within the gut or an air embolus).
- May cause bone marrow suppression by inhibiting the production of factors necessary for the synthesis of DNA. The length of exposure necessary may be as short as a few hours, and recovery usually occurs within one week.
- At the end of anaesthesia, nitrous oxide rapidly diffuses into the alveoli, reducing the partial pressure of oxygen, and can result in hypoxia (diffusion hypoxia) if the patient is breathing air. This can be overcome by increasing the inspired oxygen concentration during recovery from anaesthesia.

Malignant hyperpyrexia (hyperthermia)

Malignant hyperpyrexia (MH) is a rare, inherited disorder of skeletal muscle metabolism due to the presence of an abnormality in the ryanodine receptor in the sarcoplasmic reticulum, which results in the release of abnormally high concentrations of calcium causing increased muscle activity and metabolism. Excess heat production causes a rise in core temperature of at least 2 °C/hour. It is triggered by exposure to any of the inhalational anaesthetic drugs. For many years, suxamethonium was also considered to be a potent trigger, but recently this has been called into question. It is commoner in young adults undergoing relatively minor surgery, for example for squints, hernia repair, cleft palate repair and orthopaedic surgery. The incidence is between 1:10 000 and 1:40 000 anaesthetized patients. For more detail, refer to the guidance issued by the AAGBI [4.1].

Presentation

- An unexplained:
  - increase in end-tidal CO_2;
  - tachycardia;
  - increase in oxygen requirement (a falling SpO_2 despite increased inspired oxygen concentration).
- A progressive rise in body temperature (this may be a late sign).
- Tachypnoea in spontaneously breathing patients.
- Muscle rigidity, especially persistent masseter spasm after suxamethonium.

Immediate management

- GET HELP.
- Stop all volatile anaesthetic drugs, maintain anaesthesia with a total intravenous technique.
- Change the anaesthesia circuits and soda lime.
- Hyperventilate with 100% oxygen.
- Use a high fresh gas flow to flush the inhalational anaesthetic from the patient and machine.
- Maintain or start muscle relaxation with a non-depolarizing neuromuscular blocking drug.
- Terminate surgery as soon as practical.
- Give dantrolene 2–3 mg/kg IV, then 1 mg/kg boluses as required (up to 10 mg/kg may be needed).
- Start active cooling:
  - cold 0.9% saline IV;
  - surface cooling – ice over axillary and femoral arteries, wet sponging and fanning to encourage cooling by evaporation;
  - consider gastric or peritoneal lavage with cold saline.
- Treat acidosis with 8.4% sodium bicarbonate 50 mmol (50 mL) IV titrated to acid–base results.
- Treat hyperkalaemia.

- Transfer the patient to the intensive therapy unit (ITU) as soon as possible for:
  - temperature monitoring; may be labile for up to 48 hours;
  - continuation of dantrolene to alleviate muscle rigidity;
  - monitoring of urine output for myoglobin and treatment to prevent renal failure;
  - monitoring for and treatment of coagulopathy.

Dantrolene

This is the only specific treatment for MH. It inhibits calcium release, preventing further muscle activity. Dantrolene is orange in colour, supplied in vials containing 20 mg (plus 3 g mannitol), requires 60 mL water for reconstitution and is very slow to dissolve.

Investigation of the family

Following an episode, the patient and their family should be referred to a MH unit for investigation of their susceptibility to MH.

Anaesthesia for malignant hyperpyrexia-susceptible patients

- Employ a regional technique using plain bupivacaine if appropriate.
- General anaesthesia:
  - remove vaporizers from the anaesthetic machine;
  - use new circuits, hoses and soda lime;
  - flush the machine with high oxygen flow prior to use;
  - use total intravenous anaesthesia (TIVA) (see below); an infusion of propofol and remifentanil and oxygen-enriched air for ventilation;
  - consider pretreatment with dantrolene (orally or IV) in those who have survived a previous episode;
  - monitor temperature, ensure cooling available.

Total intravenous anaesthesia

When IV drugs alone are given to induce and maintain anaesthesia, the term 'total intravenous anaesthesia' (TIVA) is used. For a drug to be of use in maintaining anaesthesia, it must be rapidly metabolized to inactive substances or eliminated to prevent accumulation and delayed recovery, and must have no unpleasant side-effects. Currently, an infusion of propofol is the only technique used; ketamine is associated with an unpleasant recovery, and recovery after barbiturates is prolonged due to their accumulation (see Chapter 5).

Neuromuscular blocking drugs

These work by preventing acetylcholine interacting with the postsynaptic (nicotinic) receptors on the motor endplate on the skeletal muscle membrane (and possibly other sites). Muscle relaxants are divided into two groups and named to reflect what is thought to be their mode of action.

Depolarizing neuromuscular blocking drugs

Suxamethonium

This is the only drug of this type in regular clinical use. It comes ready prepared (50 mg/mL, 2 mL ampoules). The dose in adults is 1.5 mg/kg IV. After injection, there is a short period of muscle fasciculation as the muscle membrane is depolarized, followed by muscular paralysis in 40–60 seconds. Recovery occurs spontaneously as suxamethonium is hydrolysed by the enzyme plasma (pseudo-) cholinesterase, and normal neuromuscular transmission is restored after 4–6 minutes. This rapid onset makes it the drug of choice to facilitate tracheal intubation in patients likely to regurgitate and aspirate, as part of a technique called a rapid-sequence induction (RSI; see Chapter 7).

Suxamethonium has no direct effect on the cardiovascular, respiratory or central nervous systems. Bradycardia secondary to vagal stimulation is common after very large or repeated doses, and can be avoided by pretreatment with atropine. Suxamethonium has a number of important side-effects (Table 4.4).

Pseudocholinesterase deficiency

A variety of genes has been identified that are involved in plasma cholinesterase production, some of which lead to altered metabolism of suxamethonium. The most significant genotypes are:

- *normal homozygotes*: sufficient enzyme activity to hydrolyse suxamethonium in 4–6 minutes (950 per 1000 population);

Table 4.4 Important side-effects of suxamethonium.

- Malignant hyperpyrexia in susceptible patients
- Increased intraocular pressure which may cause loss of vitreous in penetrating eye injuries
- Muscular pain around the limb girdles, commonest 24 hours after administration in young adults
- Histamine release: usually localized but may cause an anaphylactic reaction
- Prolonged apnoea in patients with pseudocholinesterase deficiency (see later)
- A predictable rise in serum potassium by 0.5–0.7 mmol/L in all patients
- A massive rise in serum potassium may provoke arrhythmias in patients with:
  - burns, maximal three weeks to three months after the burn
  - denervation injury, e.g. spinal cord trauma, maximal after one week
  - muscle dystrophies, e.g. Duchenne's
  - crush injury

- *atypical heterozygotes*: slightly reduced enzyme activity levels; suxamethonium lasts 10–20 minutes (50 per 1000);
- *atypical homozygotes*: marked deficiency of active enzyme; members of this group remain apnoeic for up to 2 hours after being given suxamethonium (<1 per 1000).

Often, the presence of one of these abnormal genes is only suspected when a patient has an unexpectedly prolonged recovery following a dose of suxamethonium. Treatment of such a patient is with maintenance of anaesthesia or sedation and ventilatory support until spontaneous recovery occurs. The patient should subsequently be warned, investigated to determine their genotype and given a card that carries details. Because of its inherited nature, the remainder of the family should also be investigated.

Non-depolarizing neuromuscular blocking drugs

These drugs compete with acetylcholine and block its access to the postsynaptic receptor sites on the muscle but do not cause depolarization. (They may also block presynaptic receptors responsible for facilitating the release of acetylcholine.) The time to maximum effect, that is when relaxation is adequate to allow tracheal intubation, is relatively slow compared with suxamethonium, generally 1.5–3 minutes. A synopsis of the drugs used is given in Table 4.5.

They are used in two ways:

- following suxamethonium to maintain muscle relaxation during surgery;
- to facilitate tracheal intubation in non-urgent situations.

Although recovery of normal neuromuscular function will eventually occur spontaneously after the use of these drugs, it is often accelerated by the administration of an anticholinesterase.

Anticholinesterases

The action of all the neuromuscular blocking drugs will wear off spontaneously with time but this is not always clinically appropriate or convenient. If reversal of neuromuscular blockade due to a non-depolarizing neuromuscular blocker is required, an anticholinesterase is given (they cannot reverse the blockade induced by suxamethonium and would actually potentiate its action!). This inhibits the action of the enzyme acetylcholinesterase, leading to an increase in the concentration of acetylcholine within the synaptic cleft of the neuromuscular junction. It is accepted practice that anticholinesterases are only used once there is return of at least two twitches on peripheral nerve stimulation using the train-of-four assessment (see Chapter 3). If used in the presence of more profound neuromuscular block, there is an increased chance of residual muscle paralysis in the immediate postoperative period.

Anticholinesterases also increase the amount of acetylcholine within parasympathetic synapses (muscarinic receptors), causing bradycardia, spasm of the bowel, bladder and bronchi, increased bronchial secretions, etc. To prevent the unwanted muscarinic effects, they are always given with a suitable dose of an antimuscarinic.

The most commonly used anticholinesterase is neostigmine:

- a fixed dose of 2.5 mg intravenously is used in adults;
- its maximal effect is seen after approximately 5 minutes and lasts for 20–30 minutes;
- it is given concurrently with either atropine 1.2 mg or glycopyrrolate 0.5 mg.

Sugammadex

This is a drug that is able to reverse any intensity of neuromuscular block induced by drugs of the aminosteroid group, i.e. rocuronium and vecuronium. The dose needed and time taken for complete return of neuromuscular function vary depending on the intensity of the neuromuscular block to be reversed and range from 4 to 16 mg/kg and 1 to 3 minutes, respectively. Sugammadex works by enveloping the molecules of the neuromuscular blocker, rendering it inactive. The sugammadex-muscle relaxant complex is then excreted in the urine. Using sugammadex removes the need for, and unwanted side-effects of, both anticholinesterases and antimuscarinics when reversing residual neuromuscular block. It is not commonly used for routine reversal of neuromuscular blockade due to its cost, but it may have a role in the reversal of rocuronium-induced neuromuscular blockade in an emergency such as 'can't intubate, can't ventilate' (see later).

Analgesic drugs

Analgesic drugs are used as part of the anaesthetic technique to reduce the autonomic response to surgery, allow lower concentrations of inhalational or intravenous drugs to be given to maintain anaesthesia, and try to minimize immediate postoperative pain.

Opioid analgesics

This term is used to describe all drugs that have an analgesic effect mediated through opioid receptors, including both naturally occurring and synthetic compounds. The term 'opiate' is reserved for naturally occurring substances, such as morphine. They produce their effects at a cellular level by activating opioid receptors. These receptors are distributed throughout the central nervous system, in particular in the substantia gelatinosa of the spinal cord and the periaqueductal grey matter of the midbrain. There are several types of opioid receptors and since their identification they have had a variety of names. The current nomenclature for identification of opioid receptors is that approved by the International Union of Pharmacology: MOP, KOP, DOP and NOP receptors (previously called mu, kappa and delta opioid peptides; NOP has no previous name), each of which has a number of different subtypes.

Table 4.5 Non-depolarizing neuromuscular blocking drugs.

Drug	Dose for intubation	Maintenance dose	Time to intubation (seconds)	Clinical duration of action (minutes)	Systemic effects	Comments
Atracurium	0.5–0.6 mg/kg	0.15–0.2 mg/kg; 30–50 mg/hou infusion	90–120	40	Cutaneous histamine release, ↓ BP	Spontaneous degradation in plasma
Cisatracurium	0.1–0.15 mg/kg	0.03 mg/kg; 6–12 mg/hour infusion	120–150	50	Minimal	Single isomer of atracurium. Greater potency, longer duration of action. Minimal histamine release
Rocuronium	0.6–0.7 mg/kg. For RSI 1.0–1.2 mg/kg	0.15–0.2 mg/kg; 30–50 mg/hour infusion	60–90 after 0.6 mg/kg, 40–50 after 1.2 mg/kg	30–40 60–70	Minimal	Alternative to suxamethonium for RSI
Vecuronium	0.1 mg/kg	0.02–0.03 mg/kg; 6–10 mg/hour infusion	120–150	30–35	Minimal, no histamine release	White powder, dissolved before use
Mivacurium	0.15–0.2 mg/kg	0.1 mg/kg	150–180	15–20	Histamine released if large dose injected rapidly	Metabolized by plasma cholinesterase. Rapid recovery, reversal often unnecessary

BP, blood pressure; HR, heart rate; RSI, rapid-sequence induction.

Opioid analgesics can have pure agonist, partial agonist or mixed (agonist and antagonist) actions at the receptors.

Pure agonists

This group of drugs produces the classic effects of opioids: analgesia, euphoria, sedation, depression of ventilation and physical dependence. The systemic effects of opioids are due to both central and peripheral actions and are summarized in Table 4.6.

A synopsis of the pure agonists used in anaesthesia is given in Table 4.7. Due to the potential for abuse and diversion, there are strict rules laid out in the Misuse of Drugs Act 1971 that govern the issue and use of most opioid drugs (see later).

Overdose

Profound respiratory depression and coma due to opioids must be treated using the ABC principles described in Chapter 9. Having created a patent airway and supported ventilation using a bag-valve-mask with supplementary oxygen, the effects of the opioid can be pharmacologically reversed (antagonized). Naloxone (0.4 mg) is diluted to 5 mL with 0.9% saline and given in incremental doses of 1 mL IV (adult dosing). Analgesia will also be reversed, and careful thought must be given to continuing analgesia. The duration of action of naloxone is lees than that of morphine so the patient may redevelop signs of opioid overdose following an initial improvement, and an infusion may be needed. In this situation, monitoring in a high-dependency unit (HDU) is usually advisable.

Long-term complications of opioids

Adequate treatment of acute pain with opioids is not associated with dependency.

Tramadol

A weak agonist predominantly at MOP receptors with approximately 10% of morphine's potency. It causes the same side-effects as morphine, but in equi-analgesic doses the respiratory depression and constipation are less severe. Tramadol also blocks the reuptake of noradrenaline and 5-hydroxytryptamine (HT) within the central nervous system (CNS), thereby augmenting descending inhibitory pathways that modulate pain perception. As a result, naloxone

Table 4.6 Central and peripheral effects of opioids.

Central nervous system
Analgesia
Sedation
Euphoria
Nausea and vomiting
Pupillary constriction
Depression of ventilation:
- rate more than depth
- reduced response to carbon dioxide
Depression of vasomotor centre
Addiction (not with normal clinical use)

Respiratory system
Antitussive
Bronchospasm in susceptible patients

Cardiovascular system
Peripheral venodilatation
Bradycardia due to vagal stimulation

Urinary tract
Increased sphincter tone and urinary retention

Gastrointestinal tract
Reduced peristalsis causing:
- constipation
- delayed gastric emptying

Endocrine system
Release of ADH and catecholamines

Skin
Itching

ADH, antidiuretic hormone.

can only reverse the MOP receptor-mediated actions, providing only partial reversal. Well absorbed orally, the dose is 50–100 mg not more frequently than 4 hourly. Similar doses can be given IV or intramuscularly (IM).

Buprenorphine

This is a partial agonist, but 30 times more potent than morphine, with a longer duration of action, up to 8 hours. It is well absorbed when given sublingually. Nausea and vomiting may be severe and prolonged.

Table 4.7 The pure opioid agonists used in anaesthesia.

Drug	Route given	Dose	Speed of onset	Duration of action (minutes)	Comments
Morphine	IM	0.2–0.3 mg/kg	20–30 minutes	60–120	Also given subcutaneously, rectally, epidurally, intrathecally
	IV	0.1–0.15 mg/kg	5–10 minutes	45–60	Effective against visceral pain and pain of myocardial ischaemia. Less effective in trauma. Metabolized to morphine-6-glucuronide, a potent opioid. May cause toxicity in patients with impaired renal function (especially elderly)
Fentanyl	IV	1–3 µg/kg	2–3 minutes	20–30	Short procedures, spontaneous ventilation
		5–10 µg/kg	1–2 minutes	30–60	Long procedures, controlled ventilation
Alfentanil	IV	10 µg/kg	30–60 seconds	5–10	Short procedures. May cause profound respiratory depression
	IV infusion	0.5–2 µg/kg/minute	30–60 seconds	Infusion dependent	Long procedures, controlled ventilation
Remifentanil	IV infusion	0.1–0.3 µg/kg/minute	15–30 seconds	Infusion dependent	Major procedures. Very rapid recovery.
		C_e 1–6 ng/mL			Profound respiratory depression. Widely used in TIVA

C_e, effect site concentration ; TIVA, total intravenous anaesthesia.

Not completely reversed by naloxone (see below). It is also used in high doses in the treatment of opiate addiction; this makes postoperative analgesia a significant challenge and expert help should be sought.

Pure antagonists

The only one in common clinical use is naloxone. This has antagonist actions at all the opioid receptors, reversing all the centrally mediated effects of pure opioid agonists.

- The initial IV dose in adults is 0.1–0.4 mg, effective in less than 60 seconds and lasts 30–45 minutes.
- It has a limited effect against opioids, with partial or mixed actions, and complete reversal may require very high (10 mg) doses.
- Following a severe overdose, either accidental or deliberate, several doses or an infusion of naloxone may be required, as its duration of action is shorter than most opioids.

- Interestingly, naloxone also reverses the analgesia produced by acupuncture, suggesting that this is probably mediated in part by the release of endogenous opioids.

Regulation of opioid drugs

Some drugs have the potential for abuse and addiction, and their use in medicine is carefully regulated. The Misuse of Drugs Act 1971 relates to 'dangerous or otherwise harmful drugs', which are designated 'controlled drugs' and include the opioids [4.2]. The Act attempts to prevent the misuse of these substances by imposing a total prohibition on their manufacture, possession and supply. The Misuse of Drugs Regulations 2001 permits the use of controlled drugs in medicine [4.3]. The drugs covered by these regulations are classified into five schedules, each subject to a different level of control.

- *Schedule 1*: hallucinogenic drugs, including cannabis and lysergic acid diethylamide (LSD), which currently have no recognized therapeutic use.
- *Schedule 2*: this includes opioids, major stimulants (amphetamines and cocaine) and ketamine.
- *Schedule 3*: drugs thought less likely to be misused than those in schedule 2, including barbiturates, minor stimulants, buprenorphine, tramadol, temazepam and midazolam.
- *Schedule 4*: this is split into two parts:
  - benzodiazepines (except temazepam and midazolam), ketamine, which are recognized as having the potential for abuse;
  - anabolic and androgenic steroids, clenbuterol and growth hormones.
- *Schedule 5*: preparations which contain very low concentrations of codeine or morphine, such as cough mixtures.

Supply and custody of schedule 2 and certain schedule 3 drugs

In the operating theatre complex, these drugs are supplied by the pharmacy, usually at the signed, written request of a senior member of the nursing staff, specifying the drug and total quantity required. These drugs must be stored in a double-locked safe, cabinet or room, constructed and maintained in a way that prevents unauthorized access. A record must be kept of their use in the Controlled Drugs Register and must comply with the following requirements:

- separate parts of the register can be used for different drugs or strengths of drugs within a single class;
- the class of drug must be recorded at the head of each page;
- entries must be in chronological sequence;
- entries must be made on the day of the transaction or the next day;
- entries must be in ink or otherwise indelible;
- no cancellation, alteration or obliteration may be made;
- corrections must be accompanied by a dated footnote;
- the register must not be used for any other purpose;
- a separate register may be used for each department (each theatre);
- registers must be kept for two years after the last dated entry.

The specific details required with respect to supply of controlled drugs (for the patient) are the date of the transaction, name of person supplied (the patient's name), licence of person to be in possession (doctor's signature with name printed), amount given to the patient and the amount, if any, from the ampoule not given and destroyed. A fresh ampoule(s) must be used for each patient.

Disposal

Controlled drugs must be disposed of so that they do not cause environmental pollution and are rendered irretrievable to prevent misuse. In anaesthetic practice, this means disposing of all controlled drugs in liquid form in specially designed drug-denaturing kits, which are then incinerated.

Non-steroidal anti-inflammatory drugs (NSAIDs)

These drugs inhibit the enzyme cyclo-oxygenase (COX), therefore preventing the synthesis of prostaglandins, prostacyclins and thromboxane A2 from arachidonic acids. They have anti-inflammatory, analgesic, antipyretic actions. There are two main isoenzymes of cyclo-oxygenase: COX-1 and COX-2.

- *COX-1*: constitutive enzyme, responsible for synthesizing prostaglandins involved in protection of the integrity of the gastric mucosa, maintenance of renal blood flow, particularly when renal perfusion is compromised, platelet aggregation to reduce bleeding, and bone healing.
- *COX-2*: inducible, peripherally by surgery, trauma, endotoxins and in the CNS by pain.

The inhibition of COX-1 produces the unwanted effects, inhibition of COX-2 the desired therapeutic effects. The older NSAIDs are non-specific and associated with a greater incidence of complications, with elderly patients being particularly vulnerable. More recently, COX-2-specific NSAIDs have become available. These target only the inducible form of the enzyme and were originally thought to have a lower incidence of complications. Unfortunately, in long-term clinical use, this does not appear to be the case and some of these drugs have been associated with increased risk of stroke and myocardial infarction. Their main role now is in the short-term management

Table 4.8 Relative and absolute contraindications to the use of NSAIDs in anaesthesia.

Relative contraindications	Absolute contraindications
High risk of intraoperative bleeding, e.g. vascular surgery	Pre-existing renal dysfunction, hyperkalaemia
Concurrent use of ACE inhibitors, anticoagulants, nephrotoxic drugs	Cardiac failure
Hepatic dysfunction	Severe hepatic dysfunction
Bleeding disorders	History of GI bleeding
Elderly (>65 years)	Hypersensitivity to NSAIDs
Pregnancy and during lactation	Aspirin-induced asthma
Asthma	

ACE, angiotensin converting enzyme; GI, gastrointestinal; NSAID, non-steroidal anti-inflammatory drugs.

of acute pain. The relative and absolute contraindications to the use of these drugs are given in Table 4.8.

Parecoxib is an NSAID commonly used in the perioperative period:

- a selective COX-2 inhibitor, with predominantly analgesic activity, usually given IV but can be given IM;
- initial IV dose 40 mg, subsequent doses 20–40 mg, 6–12 hourly, maximum 80 mg/day for 2 days – reduce dose by 50% in elderly;
- effective after orthopaedic surgery, has opioid-sparing effects after abdominal surgery;
- no effect on ventilation or cardiovascular function;
- not subject to the Misuse of Drugs Regulations 2001.

Paracetamol

This has good analgesic and antipyretic properties, with little anti-inflammatory action, and is usually classified as a simple analgesic. The exact mechanism of action remains unclear, but it is thought to act on pain pathways within the CNS. It is well absorbed when taken orally, with minimal adverse effect on the gastrointestinal tract. Widely used orally for the treatment of mild-to-moderate pain in a dose of 1 g 4–6 hourly, maximum 4 g/day (lower doses are used for patients under 50 kg in weight). It is often incorporated into compound preparations with aspirin or codeine. An intravenous preparation is available containing 10 mg/mL, in 100 mL vials (1 g). The dose is the same as for the oral preparation, can be infused over 15 minutes and is effective in 5–10 minutes. It is the safest of all analgesics but patients may need reassurance that regular dosing of 1 g every 6 hours is not associated with hepatic toxicity.

Alpha-2 adrenoreceptor antagonists

There are two drugs commonly used, clonidine and dexmedetomidine, which have similar effects:

- sedation, due to a central action on adrenoreceptors;
- analgesia, due to action on the descending pathways in the dorsal horn;
- reduce blood pressure and heart rate due to an action on postsynaptic alpha-2 receptors.

Clonidine is used as an adjunct to local anaesthetics, epidurally (1–2 μg/kg in children, 75–150 μg in adults) and intrathecally (30–60 μg). It also has opioid-sparing effects when used IV, and is often used intraoperatively as an infusion (0.3–2.0 μg/kg/hour). During recovery, it can be given as a slow injection, titrated against pain and blood pressure (up to 3 μg/kg). The main side-effects are sedation, hypotension and bradycardia which are dose related. The sedative effect is sometimes used for ventilated patients in the ITU.

Dexmedetomidine is more selective than clonidine and also shorter acting. It is used in a similar way to clonidine, as an adjunct for intrathecal and peripheral nerve blocks and to provide sedation during surgical procedures performed with the patient awake and for critically ill patients in the ITU. Its effects on the cardiovascular system are also used as an adjunct to general anaesthesia surgery to allow controlled hypotension.

Gabapentinoids

This group of drugs was originally developed as anticonvulsants. Despite their name, they have no actions on GABA receptors. Their effect in treating

Table 4.9 Commonly used antiemetic drugs, dose and ideal timing.

Type of drug	Example	Usual dose	Timing	Notes
Dopamine antagonists	Metoclopramide	10 mg orally or IV	End of surgery	Prokinetic, extrapyramidal side-effects
5-hydroxytryptamine antagonists	Ondansetron	4–8 mg orally or IV	End of surgery	More effective at treating established vomiting
Antihistamines	Cyclizine	50 mg IM or IV	End of surgery	Cyclizine has anticholinergic properties. It may cause a tachycardia and postoperative delirium, particularly in the elderly. Painful when given IM
Anticholinergics	Hyoscine	1 mg transdermal patch	>4 hours before surgery	
Corticosteroid	Dexamethasone	4–8 mg IV	At induction	Causes perineal burning sensation if given to awake patients

IM, intramuscular; IV, intravenous.

acute pain is thought to come from blocking postsynaptic calcium channels and inhibiting neuronal calcium influx and pain signal transmission in the dorsal horns. This reduces the release of excitatory neurotransmitters such as glutamate and substance P from the primary afferent nerve fibres, suppressing neuronal excitability after nerve or tissue injury. They also have a role in preventing central sensitization and subsequent hyperalgesia (increased sensitivity of pain receptors to stimuli) and allodynia (pain from a stimulus not normally painful), with only minor effects on normal nociceptive pathways. They are not metabolized in humans and are eliminated unchanged in the urine. They do not induce or inhibit hepatic microsomal enzymes.

The drugs used are gabapentin and pregabalin. In acute pain, when used as part of a multimodal approach, the dose of gabapentin is 300–600 mg orally, 1–2 hours preoperatively; further doses can be given postoperatively. The dose of pregabalin is 75–300 mg orally. The most frequent side-effects of these drugs are sedation and visual disturbances.

Ketamine

In doses used to provide analgesia, ketamine blocks N-methyl-D-aspartate (NMDA) receptors in the CNS, resulting in antihyperalgesia and antiallodynia. It is usually given as an IV infusion of 0.1–0.2 mg/kg/hour,

in conjunction with an opioid and paracetamol. It is also effective against neuropathic pain. Side-effects include hallucinations, sedation and tachycardia. It is metabolized in the liver and the metabolites are excreted by the kidneys.

Antiemetics

It is not cost-effective to give antiemetic drugs to all patients and this would also potentially expose many patients to unwanted side-effects. The Apfel score (see Chapter 2) allows identification of those at greatest risk, who should receive combination therapy. Even this is not certain to prevent PONV and patients may need further treatment as they recover from anaesthesia. Some of the more commonly used antiemetic drugs are detailed in Table 4.9.

Local anaesthetic drugs

When applied to nervous tissue, these drugs cause a reversible loss of the ability to conduct nerve impulses. They can be given by a variety of routes, including topically, subcutaneously or directly adjacent to nerves.

Mechanism of action

At rest, a nerve cell has a transmembrane electrical potential (voltage) of $-70\,mV$, and is described as being 'polarized'. Noxious, mechanical, thermal or chemical stimuli, depending on their intensity, cause sodium ions (Na^+) to enter the cell. If the stimulus is of sufficient intensity, a depolarization threshold is reached that triggers sodium channels to open, allowing Na^+ to flood into the cell. As a result, the cell's membrane potential is reversed to $+20\,mV$ and an 'action potential' is initiated. This local change in the cell's membrane electrical potential causes adjacent voltage-gated sodium channels to open, altering that segment's membrane potential, propagating the action potential along the nerve. The membrane is rapidly repolarized to the resting level by loss of potassium ions (K^+) from within the cell, followed by active pumping out of Na^+ in exchange for K^+ by the Na/K ATPase pump. During repolarization, no action potential can be propagated by that section of nerve, thus ensuring unidirectional travel of action potentials. Not all stimuli are sufficient to reach the threshold, and so some will not lead to an action potential being initiated or propagated. Action potentials are 'all-or-nothing' events, and all of equal magnitude. Consequently, the strength of a nervous impulse is solely dependent on the frequency of action potentials.

In myelinated nerves, the rate of conduction is vastly increased as the action potential 'jumps' between the nodes of Ranvier, a process known as 'saltatory conduction'.

Local anaesthetic drugs work by blocking the voltage-gated sodium channels from within the nerve cell, preventing entry of sodium and subsequent depolarization so that no action potentials can be initiated or propagated.

Local anaesthetic drugs exist in two forms: ionized and unionized. When a local anaesthetic is injected, the molecules exists in the ionized form. In order to cross the cell membrane, they have to be in the unionized form. This change occurs after injection because of a relatively higher pH in tissues (7.4 compared to 6.0 in solution). However, intracellular pH is lower (7.1) and so once intracellular, a greater proportion of molecules return to their ionized form. It is this form that is attracted to, and then blocks, the sodium channels. Clearly, the degree of unionized drug will have an effect on the speed of onset. This can be further increased by using a higher concentration of the drug.

The duration of action will be determined by what proportion is protein bound; generally the greater the binding to membrane proteins, the longer the duration of action. Local blood supply will also affect the speed of removal of the drug. The degree of lipid solubility will determine potency by influencing the membrane penetration by the drug but will also result in a tendency for greater toxicity.

Following the injection of a local anaesthetic drug, there is always a predictable sequence to the onset of effects as small-diameter nerves are blocked before large-diameter ones, and unmyelinated nerves are blocked before myelinated ones. Consequently, when a regional anaesthetic technique is used, the order of onset of the block is:

- autonomic fibres – vasodilatation;
- temperature;
- pain;
- touch;
- motor – paralysis.

This accounts for the warm feeling that patients frequently notice at the onset of spinal or epidural anaesthesia, and that under some circumstances they may feel no pain but may still have some movement of their legs.

Individual drugs

Local anaesthetic drugs can be divided into two groups on the basis of their chemical structure:

- *esters*: amethocaine, benzocaine, cocaine;
- *amides*: lidocaine, bupivacaine, prilocaine.

The esters were the first drugs to be introduced into clinical practice. They are relatively more toxic, allergenic and unstable than their modern counterparts the amides. Their main use today is to provide topical anaesthesia.

Amethocaine

Available as a 4% gel (Ametop®) that is applied topically at the site of intended intravenous cannulation, and is effective in 45 minutes. More dilute solutions are available to provide topical anaesthesia of the conjunctiva.

Cocaine

Available as a paste and spray, in concentrations of 4–10%, and mainly used to provide topical anaesthesia of the nasal cavity. It has sympathomimetic properties, which are advantageous – for example, profound vasoconstriction reduces bleeding and prolongs its action, but is also responsible for its toxicity and risk of arrhythmias.

Lidocaine

A local anaesthetic commonly used in a variety of techniques including topically, by infiltration, nerve blocks, epidural and spinal anaesthesia. Consequently, it is available in a range of concentrations, 0.5–10%, to suit all situations. It is often combined with adrenaline (see later). It has a relatively fast onset and medium duration of effect. The currently accepted maximum safe dose is:

- 3 mg/kg, maximum 200 mg (without adrenaline);
- 6–7 mg/kg, maximum 500 mg (with adrenaline).

These doses should be reduced if the patient is elderly, frail or shocked. It can also be used in the treatment of ventricular fibrillation/ventricular tachycardia (VF/VT) refractory to defibrillation (100 mg IV) when amiodarone is unavailable. As with all amide local anaesthetics, it is metabolized in the liver.

Bupivacaine

Bupivacaine has a slower onset but a longer duration of action than lidocaine, and is widely used for nerve blocks, epidural and spinal anaesthesia, particularly in obstetric anaesthesia. It is available as either 0.25% or 0.5% solution, with or without adrenaline, as a hyperbaric 0.5% preservative-free solution with 8% dextrose for use in spinal anaesthesia, and as 0.1% and 0.125% solutions, which are used for epidural infusion to provide pain relief during labour and postoperatively. The current maximum safe dose is 2 mg/kg, with or without adrenaline, in any 4-hour period. Bupivacaine is significantly more cardiotoxic than other amide local anaesthetics and toxicity is difficult to treat (see Chapter 6).

Bupivacaine molecules can exist in two forms that are 'mirror images' of each other, termed stereoisomers. The two different forms of the molecule are described according to various conventions, the commonest being based upon their ability to rotate polarized light, either + or D (dextrorotatory) or – or L (laevorotatory). Bupivacaine is produced for clinical use as a racemic mixture, meaning it contains both isomers in equal quantities; levobupivacaine (Chirocaine®) is the pure L-isomer. Whichever form is used, the doses are the same, but levobupivacaine has the advantage of significantly reduced cardiotoxicity.

Ropivacaine

An amide local anaesthetic with the same potency and duration of action as bupivacaine, but lower toxicity. It also has the advantage of reduced duration and intensity of motor block, which makes it useful for postoperative analgesia.

Prilocaine

Closely related to lidocaine, prilocaine's advantages are rapid onset and reduced toxicity for a given dose. It is a component of EMLA, a cream that contains lidocaine and prilocaine in equal proportions (25 mg of each per gram). It is applied to the skin and produces surface analgesia in approximately 60 minutes. In this form, it is used to reduce the pain associated with venepuncture, particularly in children. A 2% solution of hyperbaric prilocaine has recently been introduced for spinal anaesthesia for short procedures. (A gel containing 4% amethocaine is also available for surface analgesia.)

A synopsis of the drugs used for local and regional anaesthesia is given in Table 4.10. Management of overdose and toxicity of local anaesthetic drugs are covered in Chapter 6.

Adrenaline (epinephrine)

Adrenaline is a potent vasoconstrictor as a result of its action at alpha-adrenergic receptors and is added to local anaesthetics to reduce blood flow at the site of injection. This reduces the rate of absorption, reduces toxicity and extends the duration of action. These effects are most obvious during infiltration anaesthesia and nerve blocks, and less so in epidurals or spinals. Some authorities recommend that solutions containing adrenaline should never be used intrathecally. Only very small concentrations of adrenaline are required to obtain intense vasoconstriction. The concentration of adrenaline is expressed as the weight of adrenaline (g) per volume of solution (mL). Concentrations commonly used with local anaesthetics range from 1:80 000 to 1:200 000.

Local anaesthetics containing vasoconstrictors should not be used around extremities (for example, fingers, toes, penis) because of the risk of vasoconstriction causing tissue necrosis.

The maximum safe dose of adrenaline in an adult is 250 μg, that is, 20 mL of 1:80 000 or 50 mL of 1:200 000. This should be reduced by 50% in patients with ischaemic heart disease.

Calculation of doses

For any drug, it is essential that the correct dose is given and that the maximum safe dose is never exceeded. This can be confusing with local anaesthetic drugs as

Table 4.10 Local anaesthetic drugs.

Drug	Dose	Speed of onset	Duration of action	Comments
Lidocaine	Plain: 3mg/kg, max 200mg With adrenaline: 6mg/kg, max 500mg	Rapid	60–180 minutes, depending on the technique used	Used: topically, infiltration, nerve blocks, IVRA, epidurally, intrathecally
Bupivacaine	± adrenaline: 2mg/kg, max 150mg in any 4-hour period	Nerve block: up to 40 minutes Epidurally: 15–20 minutes Intrathecal: 30 seconds	Up to 24 hours 3–4 hours, dose dependent 2–3 hours, dose dependent	Relatively cardiotoxic
Levo-bupivacaine	An isomer of bupivacaine; most properties very similar, but less cardiotoxic			This allows slightly higher doses to be given
Ropivacaine	3mg/kg, max 200mg	Similar to bupivacaine	Shorter than bupivacaine	Relatively less intense motor block than bupivacaine

IVRA, intravenous regional anaesthesia.

the volume containing the required dose will vary depending upon the concentration (expressed in percent) and a range of concentrations exists for each drug. The relationship between concentration, volume and dose is given by the formula:

$$Concentration(\%) \times Volume(mL) \times 10 = dose(mg)$$

Intravenous fluids

During anaesthesia, fluids are given intravenously to replace losses due to surgery and to provide the patient's normal daily requirements [4.4]. Three types are used: crystalloids, colloids and blood and its components.

Crystalloids

These are solutions of crystalline solids in water. The solutions can be considered in two groups: those that contain electrolytes in a similar composition to plasma, have an osmolality similar to plasma and are often referred to as being isotonic, and those that contain fewer or no electrolytes (hypotonic) but contain glucose to ensure that they have an osmolality similar to plasma. A summary of the composition of the most commonly used is shown in Table 4.11.

Once these fluids are given, they are redistributed amongst the various body fluid compartments, the extent depending on their composition. For example, 0.9% saline is distributed throughout the intravascular and interstitial volumes (extracellular fluid (ECF) compartment) in proportion to their size. After 15–30 minutes, only 25–30% of the volume administered remains intravascular. Therefore, if such a fluid is used to restore the circulating volume, 3–4 times the deficit will need to be given. If a hypotonic solution is given, for example 5% glucose, once the glucose is metabolized the remaining fluid is distributed throughout the entire body water (extracellular and intracellular volumes) and less than 10% will remain intravascular. Glucose-containing solutions are a way of treating dehydration as a result of water losses but may cause hyponatraemia. They are not routinely used perioperatively. Traditionally, 0.9% saline solution has been widely used in the perioperative period and as the first line for emergency fluid resuscitation. However, large volumes cause hyperchloraemic metabolic acidosis as, although regarded as isotonic, it contains a greater concentration of chloride than plasma.

Colloids

These are suspensions of high molecular weight particles. The most commonly used are derived from gelatin (for example, Haemaccel®, Gelofusine®) or protein (albumin). Colloids primarily expand the intravascular volume and can initially be given in a volume similar to the estimated deficit to maintain the circulating volume. However, they have a finite

Table 4.11 Composition of crystalloids.

Crystalloid	Na⁺ (mmol/L)	K⁺ (mmol/L)	Ca⁺⁺ (mmol/L)	Mg⁺⁺ (mmol/L)	Cl⁻(mmol/L)	Buffer (mmol/L)	pH	Osmolality (mosmol/L)
Hartmann's (compound sodium lactate)	131	5	4	0	112	Bicarbonate 29*	6.5	281
Plasma-Lyte®148	140	5	0	1.5	98	Acetate 27 Gluconate 23	6.5	295
0.9% sodium chloride	154	0	0	0	154	0	5.5	300
4% glucose plus 0.18% sodium chloride	31	0	0	0	31	0	4.5	284
5% glucose	0	0	0	0	0	0	4.1	278

*Present as lactate, which is metabolized to bicarbonate by the liver.

Table 4.12 Composition of colloids.

Colloid	Average molecular weight (kDa)	Na⁺ (mmol/L)	K⁺ (mmol/L)	Ca⁺⁺ (mmol/L)	Cl⁻ (mmol/L)	Buffer (mmol/L)	pH	Osmolality (mosmol/L)
Gelofusine	35	154	0.4	0.4	125	0	7.4	465
Gelaspan	26.5	151	4	1.0	103	Acetate (24)	7.4	284
Isoplex 4%*	30	145	4	(Mg⁺⁺ 0.9)	105	Lactate (25)	7.4	284
Haemaccel	35	145	5	6.2	145	0	7.3	350
Albumin	69	130–160	2	0	120	0	6.7–7.3	270–300

*Calcium replaced with magnesium.

life in the plasma and will eventually be either metabolized or excreted, and therefore need replacing. A summary of their composition is shown in Table 4.12. There is no limit on the volume of gelatins that can be given (provided that haemoglobin concentration is maintained!); however, of the colloids, they have the greatest tendency to release histamine and may rarely cause anaphylaxis (1–2 cases per 10000 units given). In 2014, the MHRA restricted the use of starch products and they are now no longer permitted in patients with sepsis, burn injuries or the critically ill because of an increased risk of renal failure and mortality. They are only indicated for the treatment of hypovolaemia, due to acute blood loss when crystalloids alone are not considered sufficient. They should not be used for more than 24 hours, up to a maximum volume of 30 mL/kg, and renal function must be monitored for at least 90 days. As a result, the use of starch solutions has virtually ceased. Recently, there has been an increase in the use of 4–5% human albumin solution, particularly in patients in critical care.

Blood and blood components

Before use, donated whole blood is generally processed into the following products to allow the most appropriate components to be given [4.5].

- *Red cells in optimal additive solution (SAG-M)*: a red cell concentrate to which a mixture of saline, adenine and glucose and mannitol has been added. This improves both red cell survival and flow characteristics. Each unit contains approximately 300 mL with a haematocrit of 50–70% and will raise a patient's haemoglobin by roughly 1 g/dL. White cells are routinely removed in the UK to prevent the risk of prion disease transmission.
- *Platelet concentrates*: supplied either as 'units' containing 50–60 mL (55×10^9 platelets) or as bags equivalent to four units. Four units or one bag will raise the platelet count by $30–40 \times 10^9$/L. It is given via a standard giving set **without** the use of a microaggregate filter, as this will result in the loss of significant numbers of platelets.
- *Fresh frozen plasma (FFP)*: one unit consists of the plasma separated from a single donation, usually 200–250 mL, and frozen within 6 hours. It contains normal levels of clotting factors (except factor VIII, 70% normal). An adult dose is four units. It should be infused as soon as it has thawed.
- *Cryoprecipitate*: on controlled thawing of FFP, a precipitate is formed, which is collected and suspended in plasma. It contains large amounts of factor VIII and fibrinogen. It is supplied as a pooled donation from six packs of FFP in one unit and must be used as soon as possible after thawing.

Details of fluid management can be found in Chapter 5 (intraoperative) and Chapter 8 (postoperative).

Risks of blood and blood product transfusions

All blood donations are routinely tested for hepatitis B surface antigen, hepatitis C, syphilis, human T-cell lymphotrophic virus (HTLV), and antibodies to HIV. However, a period exists between exposure to viruses and the development of antibodies, during which the infected red cells would not be detected by current screening techniques. The risk is very small, and has been estimated for hepatitis B at $1:10^5$ and for HIV at $1:10^6$ units transfused.

In order to try to eliminate these risks, techniques now exist for using the patient's own blood in the perioperative period. This also has the advantage of reducing the chances of, but not eliminating, the wrong unit of blood being transfused [4.6].

- *Predepositing blood*: over a period of four weeks prior to surgery, the patient builds up a bank of 2–4 units of blood for retransfusion perioperatively.
- *Preoperative haemodilution*: following induction of anaesthesia, 0.5–1.5 L of blood is removed and replaced with colloid. This can then be transfused at the end of surgery.
- *Cell savers*: these devices collect blood lost during surgery via a suction system; the red cells are separated, washed and resuspended, ready for retransfusion to the patient (see Chapter 2).

FURTHER INFORMATION

British Medical Association and the Royal Pharmaceutical Society of Great Britain. British National Formulary (BNF). London: British Medical Association and the Royal Pharmaceutical Society of Great Britain. www.medicinescomplete.com/mc/bnf/current/

Hopkins PM. Malignant hyperthermia: pharmacology of triggering. British Journal of Anaesthesia 2011; 107: 48–56.

Peck TE, Hill SA, Williams M (eds). Pharmacology for Anaesthesia and Intensive Care, 4th edn. New York: Cambridge University Press, 2014.

[4.1] www.aagbi.org/sites/default/files/MH%20guideline%20for%20web%20v2.pdf aagbi guidelines for treatment of malignant hyperthermia, 2011.

[4.2] www.dhsspsni.gov.uk/articles/misuse-drugs-legislations Law governing the use and misuse of drugs in the UK.

[4.3] www.legislation.gov.uk/uksi/2001/3998/pdfs/uksi_20013998_en.pdf Regulations regarding the supply and use of controlled drugs in medicine.

[4.4] www.nice.org.uk/guidance/cg174 The full National Institute for Health and Care Excellence (NICE) guidance on intravenous fluid therapy in adults in hospital.

[4.5] www.aagbi.org/sites/default/files/bloodtransfusion06.pdf AAGBI guidelines on blood transfusion and component therapy, 2005.

[4.6] www.shotuk.org/Serious Hazards of Transfusion (SHOT). Contains the latest UK data.

5

The practice of general anaesthesia

Learning objectives

After reading this chapter you should understand the principles of:

- ☐ The preoperative checking of the anaesthetic machine and patient
- ☐ How to establish and maintain a patent airway in an unconscious patient
- ☐ How to insert a supraglottic airway
- ☐ Direct laryngoscopy and tracheal intubation
- ☐ The different components of general anaesthesia, both inhalational and TIVA
- ☐ How to position a patient safely for surgery
- ☐ Intraoperative fluid requirements
- ☐ Safe emergence from anaesthesia
- ☐ The importance of non-technical skills during anaesthesia and surgery

Apply this knowledge when practising the following skills:

- ☐ Checking a patient before the start of anaesthesia
- ☐ Inserting an IV cannula
- ☐ Using a facemask and basic adjuncts to maintain a patent airway and ventilate an unconscious patient
- ☐ Inserting a supraglottic airway device
- ☐ Performing direct laryngoscopy and tracheal intubation
- ☐ Confirming the correct positioning of a tracheal tube

There should be a smooth, controlled sequence of preplanned events from the time patients arrive in the anaesthetic room until they leave [5.1]. This chapter outlines how, by applying the knowledge and skills from the previous chapters, along with good non-technical skills, the anaesthetist achieves this and minimizes the risks of both anaesthesia and surgery [5.2]. The descriptions given follow as closely as possible the sequence of events as they might be expected to occur during anaesthesia for an elective surgical procedure.

Clinical Anaesthesia: Lecture Notes, Fifth Edition. Matthew Gwinnutt and Carl Gwinnutt.
© 2017 John Wiley & Sons, Ltd. Published 2017 by John Wiley & Sons, Ltd.
Companion website: www.lecturenoteseries.com/anaesthesia

Preoperative checks

Checking the anaesthetic machine

It is the responsibility of every anaesthetist to check the anaesthetic machine, monitors, breathing system and any ancillary equipment at the beginning of each operating session to ensure that they all function in the manner expected. The main danger is that the anaesthetic machine appears to perform normally but in fact is delivering a hypoxic mixture to the patient. Most modern integrated anaesthesia machines perform a 'self-test' when first switched on and do not need to be retested by the user. A check of the gas supply and of the breathing system for patency and lack of gas leaks is essential. The function, calibration and alarm settings on the monitors should also be checked. The AAGBI publishes a document entitled *Checking Anaesthetic Equipment* that gives more comprehensive details [5.3]. A record should be kept of each check of the anaesthetic machine and equipment. Appropriate procedures must also be in place to deal safely with any problems that are identified.

Checking the patient

Anaesthesia and surgery are not without risk. The World Health Organization (WHO) has reported that in industrialized countries, major complications occur in 3–16% of inpatient surgical procedures and permanent disability or death in 0.4–0.8%. To try and reduce this incidence of harm, a surgical safety checklist is now routinely used [5.4]. It is completed in three stages:

- before the induction of anaesthesia ('sign in');
- before the start of the surgical intervention (skin incision or equivalent) ('time out');
- before the team leaves the operating theatre (or at skin closure or its equivalent) ('sign out').

Sign in

1 When the patient arrives in the anaesthetic room, the anaesthetist and the anaesthetist's assistant must confirm the patient's identity, usually with the patient, the patient's wrist-band and case notes. The nature of the planned operation, site and side (if appropriate) are confirmed with the patient and a check is made to ensure the correct surgical site is clearly marked. The consent form is checked to ensure the correct details are entered and the patient and surgical team have signed it appropriately. When the patient is unable to confirm their details, for example a ventilated intensive care patient, great care should be taken and the above checks performed preferably by both the anaesthetist and surgeon.

2 A record is made that the anaesthetic machine has been checked along with the drugs required for the case.

3 A specific check is made of any known allergies the patient may have.

4 A specific check is made to ensure that any anticipated or known problems with airway management have been identified and equipment is available.

5 Anticipated blood loss and availability of blood are checked.

 KEY POINT

- A formal check of the identity, operation, side/site and consent form **must** be made by the anaesthetist and surgeon before every operation.

Preparation for anaesthesia

Several things now happen, often simultaneously:

- monitoring equipment is attached to the patient;
- IV access is obtained;
- the patient is preoxygenated.

Once all of these have been achieved satisfactorily, the patient is anaesthetized.

Monitoring the patient

This should commence before the induction of anaesthesia and continue until the patient has recovered from the effects of anaesthesia, and the information generated should be recorded in the patient's notes, either written or electronically. The type and number of monitors used depend upon a variety of factors, including:

- type of operation and operative technique;
- anaesthetic technique used;

- present and previous health of the patient;
- equipment available and the anaesthetist's ability to use it;
- preferences of the anaesthetist;
- any research being undertaken.

The AAGBI has identified certain monitoring devices as *essential* for the safe conduct of anaesthesia. These are electrocardiogram (ECG), non-invasive blood pressure (NIBP), pulse oximeter, capnography and vapour concentration analysis. Clearly, the latter two are only used after general anaesthesia has commenced. In addition, a peripheral nerve stimulator should be **immediately available**. Finally, additional monitoring equipment will be required in certain cases, for example invasive blood pressure, urine output, central venous pressure (CVP) and various haemodynamic parameters [3.5].

NICE guidelines recommend that all patients should have their temperature measured before induction of anaesthesia, and surgery should not be started (unless there is a critical need) if it is below 36 °C. Subsequently the patient's temperature should be measured every 30 minutes [3.7]. Active warming should be used as described below.

If depth of anaesthesia monitoring, e.g. bispectral index (BIS), is being planned then it is also applied at this point; intubation (especially difficult intubation), transfer into theatre and skin incision are some of the times when patients are most at risk of accidental awareness (see Chapter 3).

There is good evidence that monitoring reduces the risks of adverse incidents and accidents. The combination of pulse oximetry, capnography and blood pressure monitoring will detect the majority of serious incidents early and before there has been serious harm to the patient. Ultimately, monitoring supplements clinical observation; there is no substitute for the presence of a trained and experienced anaesthetist throughout the entire operative procedure.

Monitoring is not without its own potential hazards:

- faulty equipment may endanger the patient, for example from electrocution secondary to faulty earthing;
- the anaesthetist may act on faulty data, instituting inappropriate treatment;
- the patient may be harmed by the complications of the technique to establish invasive monitoring, for example pneumothorax following central venous catheterization.

Ultimately, an excessive number of monitors may distract the anaesthetist from observation of the patient and compromise their situational awareness.

 KEY POINT

- Essential and appropriate monitoring **must** be used in every patient who undergoes anaesthesia.

Intravenous access

The superficial veins on the back of the hand (dorsal metacarpal veins) and forearm (cephalic and basilic veins) are most commonly used for IV access. Veins in the antecubital fossa tend to be used either in an emergency situation or when attempts to cannulate peripheral veins have failed. It must be remembered that the brachial artery, the median nerve and branches of the medial and lateral cutaneous nerves of the arm are in close proximity to the antecubital veins and easily damaged by needles or extravasated drugs. A cannula must not be sited in the arm on the side where the patient has either undergone clearance of axillary lymph nodes for malignant disease or has had a fistula for dialysis created. The former increases the risk of exacerbating lymphoedema and in the latter, the fistula may be damaged. Peripheral venous cannulation is an essential skill, best learnt under the supervision of an anaesthetist, rather than reading about it! Complications of peripheral venous cannulation are shown in Table 5.1.

The size of cannula inserted will depend upon its purpose: large-diameter cannulas (14 G or 2.0 mm, 16 G or 1.8 mm) are required for giving fluid rapidly; smaller ones (20 G or 1.0 mm) are adequate for giving drugs and maintenance fluids. When inserting a large cannula prior to induction of anaesthesia, a small amount of local anaesthetic (0.2 mL lidocaine 1%) should be infiltrated into the skin at the site chosen for venepuncture using a 25 G (0.5 mm) needle. This reduces pain and makes the patient less likely to move and less resistant to further attempts.

As with any procedure where there is a risk of contact with body fluids, gloves must always be worn by the operator.

Central venous cannulation

This is used to allow monitoring of the cardiovascular system or to give certain drugs (for example, inotropes) and cannulation is usually performed after the patient has been anaesthetized. Rarely, it may be required before anaesthesia is induced because of a lack of or inadequate peripheral venous access (for

Table 5.1 Complications of peripheral venous cannulation.

- *Failure*: attempt cannulation distally in a limb and work proximally. If multiple attempts are required, fluid or drugs will not leak from previous puncture sites.
- *Haematoma*: usually secondary to the above with inadequate pressure applied over the puncture site to prevent bleeding, and made worse by forgetting to remove the tourniquet!
- *Extravasation of fluid or drugs*: failing to recognize that the cannula is not within the vein before use. May cause damage to the surrounding tissues.
- *Damage to local structures*: secondary to poor technique and lack of knowledge of the local anatomy.
- *Air embolus*: most likely following cannulation of a central vein (see below).
- *Shearing of the cannula*: usually a result of trying to reintroduce the needle after it has been withdrawn. The safest action is to withdraw the whole cannula and attempt again at another site.
- *Thrombophlebitis*: related to the length of time the vein is in use and irritation caused by the substances flowing through it. High concentrations of drugs and fluids with extremes of pH or high osmolality are the main causes, e.g. antibiotics, calcium chloride, sodium bicarbonate. Once a vein shows signs of thrombophlebitis (i.e. tender, red and deteriorating flow), the cannula must be removed to prevent subsequent infection or thrombosis.

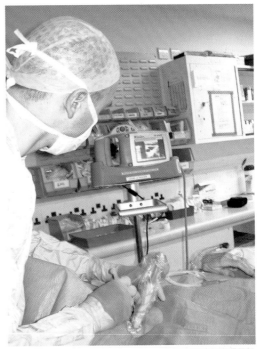

(a)

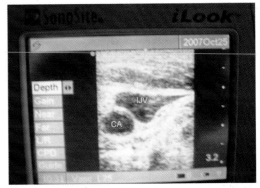

(b)

Figure 5.1 (a) CVP catheter being inserted using ultrasound guidance. (b) Ultrasound screen showing relative positions of the internal jugular vein (IJV) and carotid artery (CA).

example, in a patient who has a history of IV drug abuse). It is included at this point for completeness. There are many different types of equipment and approaches to the central veins, and the following is intended as an outline. It is now recommended that an ultrasound scanner is used to detect the internal jugular vein and guide the insertion of the needle into the vein [5.5] (Figure 5.1).

Internal jugular vein

This approach is associated with the highest incidence of success (95%), and a low rate of complications (Table 5.2). The right internal jugular offers certain advantages: there is a 'straight line' to the heart, the apical pleura does not rise as high on this side and the main thoracic duct is on the left.

Subclavian vein

This can be approached by both the supra- and infra-clavicular routes. Both are technically more difficult than the internal jugular route and there is a significant risk of causing a pneumothorax (approximately 2%). The main advantages of this route are comfort for the patient and low risk of infection during long-term use.

Table 5.2 Complications of internal jugular vein cannulation.

- Arterial puncture causing a haematoma or haemothorax
- Air embolus
- Venous thrombosis
- Pneumothorax
- Thoracic duct injury (left side) and chylothorax
- Hydrothorax if the catheter is intrapleural and fluid given
- Bacteraemia
- Septicaemia
- Soft tissue infection at puncture site
- Injury to nerves:
  - ○ brachial plexus
  - ○ recurrent laryngeal
  - ○ phrenic

Bilateral attempts at central venous cannulation must not be made because of the risk of haematoma formation in the neck, causing airway obstruction, or causing bilateral pneumothoraces.

Femoral vein

Often used in emergency situations, for example hypotensive trauma patients and on the intensive therapy unit (ITU) for haemofiltration. The main advantages of using this vein are that it is away from monitors and airway devices and it eliminates the possibility of a haemothorax or pneumothorax. Previously there have been concerns about the increased risk of catheter-related bloodstream infections when using this approach, but providing full aseptic precautions are taken, rates are now comparable to other sites. As with internal jugular vein cannulation, ultrasound guidance is used to identify the vein and guide the insertion of the needle into the vein.

Technique of central venous catheterization

The Seldinger technique is most commonly used for percutaneous cannulation of the central veins.

- The vein is punctured initially percutaneously using a small-diameter needle. A flexible guide-wire is then passed through the needle into the vein and the needle is carefully withdrawn, leaving the wire behind. The catheter is now passed over

the wire into the vein, usually preceded by a dilator. The operator must ensure they have hold of the wire at all times and that it is removed once the cannula is fully inserted. The advantage of this method is that the initial use of a small needle increases the chance of successful venepuncture and reduces the risk of damage to the vein.

 KEY POINT

- Whenever an internal jugular or subclavian vein central venous catheter is inserted, a chest X-ray must be taken to ensure that the catheter is correctly positioned with the tip at the junction of the superior vena cava and right atrium and that a pneumothorax has not been caused.

Arterial cannulation

This can be performed under local anaesthesia before the patient is anaesthetized or once the patient has been anaesthetized. The radial artery is most commonly used (femoral and brachial are also used) as it is superficial, compressible and there is usually good collateral circulation to the hand via the ulnar artery. It has been advocated that Allen's test to check the adequacy of the ulnar circulation is performed before radial artery cannulation.

Technique of cannulation

The wrist is fully supinated and dorsiflexed about 60°, often over a small support. The skin is cleansed appropriately and the position of the radial artery identified by palpation at the level of the proximal wrist skin crease. If local anaesthetic is used, a small volume (0.2 mL) is injected using a 25 G needle over and to either side of the artery. Two techniques are used to cannulate the artery.

- *Direct puncture* using a catheter over needle, either a non-ported IV cannula or a specifically designed arterial cannula with a built-in on/off switch. The skin is punctured at an angle of 20–30° and the needle point advanced towards the artery. As the artery is punctured, arterial blood fills the flashback chamber. The needle should then be lowered to about 10° and advanced a further 1–2 mm to ensure the tip of the cannula lies within the artery. The cannula is then advanced off the needle into the artery.

- *Seldinger technique*: the artery is punctured directly with the needle as described above. Successful puncture is confirmed by getting pulsatile blood from the hub of the needle. The guidewire is advanced through the needle and the needle carefully withdrawn, leaving the wire behind. The catheter is now passed over the wire into the artery before removal of the wire.

Once the cannula is in place, it is usually sutured to reduce the risk of accidental removal and covered with a transparent, sterile dressing.

Complications of arterial cannulation include bleeding, infection, thrombosis and aneurysm formation.

Preoxygenation

At the end of expiration, the lungs contain a significant volume of air (the functional residual capacity, FRC). The vast majority of this (~80%) is nitrogen which helps to prevent the alveoli from collapsing because it is not absorbed into the blood. The oxygen content acts as a reservoir to ensure a constant availability during the ventilatory cycle and also prevent hypoxaemia during brief periods of breath-holding. The purpose of preoxygenation is to replace the nitrogen with oxygen, thereby significantly increasing the length of time a patient can be apnoeic (or not ventilated) without becoming hypoxic, effectively 'buying time' for both the patient and anaesthetist in case of difficulty. Preoxygenation is usually achieved by getting the patient to breathe 100% oxygen via a close-fitting facemask for about three minutes or until the oxygen concentration in expired gas exceeds 85%. In an emergency situation, a reasonable degree of preoxygenation can be achieved by asking a cooperative patient to take four vital capacity breaths of 100% oxygen via an anaesthetic circuit with a tight-sealing facemask.

Induction of anaesthesia

Intravenous drugs are the most frequently used method of inducing anaesthesia. The drug dose is calculated, taking into account the patient's age and any comorbidities, and then given over 20–30 seconds. This method is generally preferred by the patient, as consciousness is lost rapidly, and by the anaesthetist because pharyngeal reflexes are depressed, allowing the insertion of an airway device. There are a number of potential disadvantages.

- Patients often become apnoeic. This may necessitate manual ventilation until spontaneous ventilation resumes.
- There may be a degree of hypotension. This will depend on the drug, dose used, speed given and 'fitness' of the patient.
- There may be loss of airway patency. This can usually be overcome by a combination of basic airway opening manoeuvres, insertion of an oropharyngeal airway or supraglottic airway (SGA) device.

Inhalational induction of anaesthesia is an alternative. A gradually increasing concentration of an inhalational drug in oxygen or a mixture of oxygen and nitrous oxide is breathed by the patient. Its advantages are that it can be used in:

- patients with a lack of suitable veins. Rather than subject the patient to repeated attempts at venepuncture, anaesthesia is induced and, as most volatile anaesthetics are vasodilators, venepuncture is then possible;
- an uncooperative child, or patients with a needle phobia. Venous access can be obtained after induction;
- patients with airway compromise, in which an IV drug may cause apnoea and loss of airway patency. Ventilation and oxygenation become impossible, with catastrophic results. Inhalation induction preserves spontaneous ventilation and if airway patency is threatened, further uptake of anaesthetic is prevented, limiting the problem.

Potential disadvantages include the following.

- Unconsciousness occurs more slowly than with an IV drug.
- Most inhalational drugs are unpleasant to breathe. Currently, sevoflurane is the only anaesthetic used for this technique.
- Hypotension and a fall in cardiac output occur with increasing concentrations. This may be difficult to treat until IV access is obtained.
- The combination of hypercapnia, as a result of respiratory depression, and the vasodilator effect of these drugs leads to increased cerebral blood flow, making this technique unsuitable in patients with raised intracranial pressure.
- It can still lead to airway obstruction, inability to ventilate and no way to exhale the anaesthetic already inhaled!

As the concentration of inhalational drug increases, there is progressive reduction in the ventilatory activity of the intercostal muscles, muscle tone generally is also reduced and laryngeal reflexes are lost. The pupils start by becoming dilated, then slightly constricted and finally gradually dilate. This point is referred to as 'surgical anaesthesia'. Any further increase in depth of anaesthesia will result in diaphragmatic paralysis and cardiovascular collapse.

As well as the above, the anaesthetic will have effects on all of the other body systems, which will need appropriate monitoring.

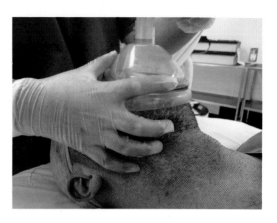

Figure 5.3 Mask being held on patient's face. Note the use of the little finger to apply a jaw thrust.

Maintaining the airway

General anaesthesia frequently causes the patient's airway to become obstructed following loss of tone in the muscles of the tongue and pharynx (Figure 5.2).

The easiest way to restore patency is through basic airway manoeuvres – a combination of the head tilt, chin lift and jaw thrust (Figure 5.3). Although a patent airway can be maintained for the duration of surgery in the majority of patients in this manner, it is increasingly uncommon as it severely restricts any further activity by the anaesthetist. This problem has been overcome by the use of a supraglottic airway device. The best method of providing and securing a clear airway in patients is tracheal intubation, but this is not appropriate in all patients.

Facemasks

A facemask is used to ensure that the anaesthetic gas mixture is delivered to the patient. Leakage of gases is minimized by using one that provides a good seal. When holding a facemask in position with the index finger and thumb, the jaw thrust is achieved by lifting the angle of the mandible with the remaining fingers of one or both hands. The overall desired effect is that the patient's mandible is 'lifted' into the mask, rather than the mask being pushed into the face (see Figure 5.3). The patient can now breathe spontaneously or be ventilated. Sometimes despite this technique, a patent airway cannot be established and additional adjuncts are needed.

Oropharyngeal airway

Estimate the size required by comparing the airway length with the vertical distance between the patient's incisor teeth (or if edentulous, the front of the mouth) and the angle of the jaw. Then insert the airway, initially 'upside down', as far as the back of the hard palate before rotating it 180° and fully inserting until the flange lies in front of the teeth (or gums in an edentulous patient) (Figure 5.4).

Nasopharyngeal airway

Choose an appropriately sized airway, 7 mm for women, 8 mm for men, check the patency of the nostril to be used (usually the right) and lubricate the airway. The airway is then inserted along the floor of the nose, with the bevel facing medially to avoid catching

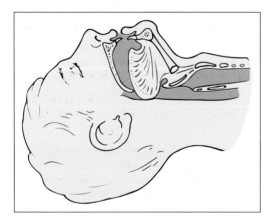

Figure 5.2 Sagittal section of the head and neck showing how the tongue contributes to airway obstruction.

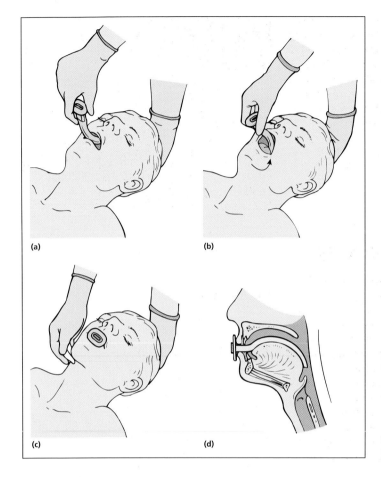

(a)

(b)

(c)

(d)

Figure 5.4 (a–d) The sequence for inserting an oropharyngeal airway.

the turbinates (Figure 5.5). A safety pin may be inserted through the flange to prevent inhalation of the airway. If obstruction is encountered, do not use force as severe bleeding may be provoked. Instead, try the other nostril.

Problems with airways

- Although the techniques described so far will create and maintain a patent airway, they offer no protection against aspiration of regurgitated gastric contents.
- Failure to maintain a patent airway: snoring, indrawing of the supraclavicular, suprasternal and intercostal spaces, use of the accessory muscles or paradoxical respiratory movement (see-saw respiration) suggest obstruction.
- Inability to maintain a good seal between the patient's face and the mask, particularly in those without teeth.
- Fatigue, when holding the mask for prolonged periods.

- The anaesthetist not being free to deal with any other problems that may arise.

These problems may be overcome by either a supraglottic airway or tracheal intubation.

Supraglottic airway devices

These are widely used in spontaneously breathing patients as they overcome some of the problems associated with the techniques described above.

- They are not affected by the shape of the patient's face or the absence of teeth.
- The anaesthetist is not required to hold them in position or maintain a jaw thrust or chin lift, thereby avoiding fatigue and allowing any other problems to be dealt with.
- They significantly reduce the risk of aspiration of regurgitated gastric contents but do not eliminate it completely.

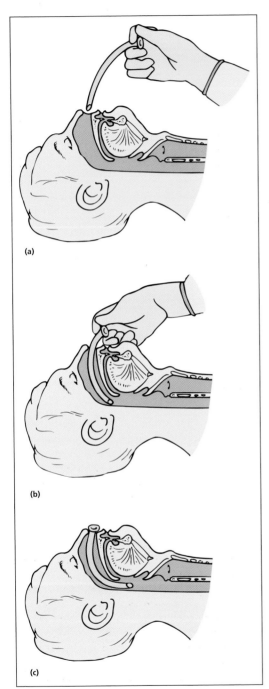

(a)

(b)

(c)

Figure 5.5 (a–c) The sequence for inserting a nasopharyngeal airway.

- Their use **is relatively contraindicated** where there is an increased risk of regurgitation, for example in emergency cases, pregnancy and patients with a hiatus hernia.

In addition to the above, these devices have proved to be a valuable aid in those patients who are difficult to intubate, as they can usually be inserted to facilitate oxygenation while additional help or equipment is obtained (see later).

Insertion of a supraglottic airway (Figure 5.6)

The technique for insertion of a laryngeal mask airway (LMA) is described, but the principles apply to all supraglottic devices, although not all have an inflatable cuff. The patient's reflexes must be suppressed to a level similar to that required for the insertion of an oropharyngeal airway to prevent coughing or laryngospasm.

- The cuff is deflated (Figure 5.6a) and the mask lightly lubricated.
- A head tilt is performed, the patient's mouth opened fully and the tip of the mask inserted along the hard palate with the open side facing but not touching the tongue (Figure 5.6b).
- The mask is further inserted, using the index finger to provide support for the tube (Figure 5.6c). Eventually, resistance will be felt at the point where the tip of the mask lies at the upper oesophageal sphincter (Figure 5.6d).
- The cuff is now fully inflated using an air-filled syringe attached to the valve at the end of the pilot tube (Figure 5.6e).
- The laryngeal mask is secured by either a length of bandage or adhesive strapping attached to the protruding tube.
- A 'bite block' may be inserted to reduce the risk of damage to the LMA at recovery.

Tracheal intubation

This requires abolition of the laryngeal reflexes. During anaesthesia, this is achieved by giving a neuromuscular blocking drug. Alternatively, deep inhalational anaesthesia or local anaesthesia of the larynx can be used, but these are generally reserved for patients in whom difficulty with intubation is anticipated, for example in the presence of airway tumours or immobility of the cervical spine. The common indications for tracheal intubation are shown in Table 5.3.

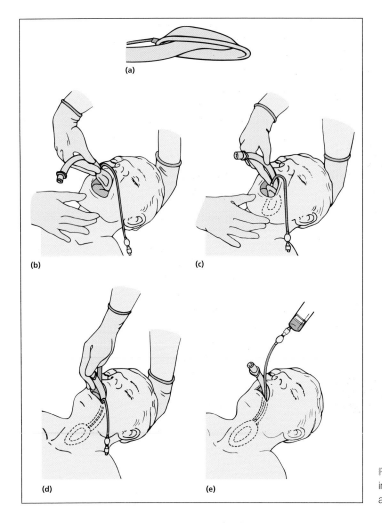

Figure 5.6 (a–e) Sequence for the insertion of a cuffed supraglottic airway device.

 KEY POINT

- Before every intubation, the anaesthetic team MUST devise and discuss the plan that will be implemented in the event of encountering difficulty to ensure that the patient does not come to harm from hypoxia.

Equipment for tracheal intubation

The equipment used will be determined by the circumstances and by the preferences of the individual anaesthetist. The following is a list of the basic needs for **adult oral** intubation.

- *Laryngoscope* with a curved (Macintosh) blade and functioning light.
- *Tracheal tubes (cuffed)* in a variety of sizes. The internal diameter is expressed in millimetres and the length in centimetres. They may be lightly lubricated.
- *For males*: 8–9 mm internal diameter, 22–24 cm length.
- *For females*: 7–8 mm internal diameter, 20 cm length.
- *Syringe* to inflate the cuff once the tube is in place.
- *Catheter mount*: to connect the tube to the anaesthetic system or ventilator tubing.
- *Suction*: switched on and immediately to hand in case the patient vomits or regurgitates.

Table 5.3 Common indications for tracheal intubation.

- Where muscle relaxants are used to facilitate surgery (e.g. abdominal and thoracic surgery), thereby necessitating the use of mechanical ventilation.
- In patients with a full stomach, to protect against aspiration.
- Where the position of the patient would make airway maintenance difficult, e.g. the lateral or prone position.
- Where there is competition between surgeon and anaesthetist for the airway (e.g. operations on the head and neck).
- Where controlled ventilation is utilized to improve surgical access (e.g. neurosurgery).
- In those patients in whom the airway cannot be satisfactorily maintained by any other technique.
- During cardiopulmonary resuscitation.

- *Capnometer*: to detect carbon dioxide in expired gas (see later), thereby confirming placement of the tube in the airway.
- *Stethoscope*: to check ventilation of both lungs is occurring by listening for breath sounds during ventilation.
- *Extras*: a semi-rigid introducer to help mould the tube to a particular shape; Magill's forceps, designed to reach into the pharynx to remove debris or direct the tip of a tube; different sizes or styles of laryngoscope blade (for example, McCoy), bandage or tape to secure the tube.

Technique of oral intubation

Following IV induction, some anaesthetists advocate ensuring that the patient can be ventilated via a face-mask before giving the neuromuscular blocking drug to facilitate intubation. If intubation then proves to be unexpectedly difficult or impossible, the anaesthetist knows that oxygenation can be maintained and the patient will come to no harm. Along with the neuromuscular blocking drug, an IV opioid is often given to reduce the cardiovascular response to intubation. During the time it takes for a non-depolarizing neuromuscular blocker to reach maximal effect, there will be a period of apnoea. The patient will need to be ventilated manually with a mixture of oxygen and an inhalational drug to maintain anaesthesia. Once the degree of neuromuscular block is adequate, direct laryngoscopy is performed.

With the patient's head on a small pillow, the neck is flexed and the head extended at the atlanto-occipital joint, in the 'sniffing the morning air' position. The patient's mouth is fully opened using the index finger and thumb of the **right** hand in a scissor action. The laryngoscope is held in the **left** hand and the blade introduced into the mouth along the right-hand side of the tongue, displacing it to the left. The blade is advanced until the tip lies in the gap between the base of the tongue and the epiglottis – the vallecula. Force is then applied **in the direction in which the handle of the laryngoscope is pointing**. The effort comes from the upper arm, not the wrist, to lift the tongue and epiglottis. This exposes the larynx, seen as a tri-angular opening with the apex anteriorly and the whitish coloured true vocal cords laterally (Figure 5.7).

The tracheal tube is introduced into the right side of the mouth, advanced and seen to pass through the cords until the cuff lies just below them. The tube is then held firmly, the laryngoscope is carefully removed and the cuff is inflated sufficiently to prevent any leak during ventilation. The patient is now ventilated manually while the position of the tube is confirmed, and it is secured to the patient using adhesive tape or cotton tape.

For some types of surgery, such as oral surgery, nasotracheal intubation is used so that the tube is out of the surgical field. A well-lubricated tube is introduced, usually via the right nostril, along the floor of the nose with the bevel pointing medially to avoid damage to the turbinates. It is advanced into the oro-pharynx, where it is usually visualized using a laryngoscope in the manner described above. It can then either be advanced directly into the larynx by pushing on the proximal end or the tip picked up with Magill's forceps (which are designed not to impair the view of the larynx) and directed into the larynx. The procedure then continues as for oral intubation.

Confirming the position of the tracheal tube

Every tracheal tube inserted **must** have its position confirmed. This can be achieved using a number of techniques of varying reliability.

- *Measuring the carbon dioxide in expired gas (waveform capnography)*: the presence of carbon dioxide in expired gas indicates that the tube is in the airway; less than 0.2% indicates oesophageal intubation. However, it does not indicate when the tube has been inserted too far and lies in a main bronchus. This can usually be determined by listening to both sides of the chest for equality of breath sounds.

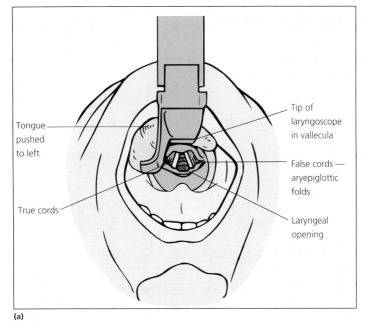

(a)

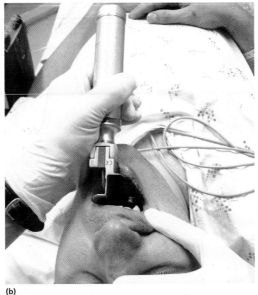

(b)

Figure 5.7 (a) Diagrammatic representation of the ideal view of the larynx at laryngoscopy. (b) Photograph showing tip of epiglottis during laryngoscopy.

- *Direct visualization*: observing the tracheal tube passing between the vocal cords.
- *Fogging*: seen on clear plastic tube connectors during expiration.
- Less reliable signs are:
  - diminished breath sounds on auscultation;
  - decreased chest movement on ventilation;
  - gurgling sounds over the epigastrium and 'burping' sounds as gas escapes;
  - a decrease in oxygen saturation detected by pulse oximetry. This occurs late, particularly if the patient has been preoxygenated.

KEY POINT

- Every patient who is intubated MUST have waveform capnography used to confirm that the tube is within the patient's airway.

Complications of tracheal intubation

The following complications are the commoner ones, not an attempt to identify all eventualities.

Hypoxia

This may be due to the following.

- *Unrecognized oesophageal intubation*: this is most likely to occur when waveform capnography is unavailable. If there is any doubt about the position of the tube, it should be removed and the patient ventilated via a facemask.
- *Failed intubation and inability to ventilate the patient*: this is a rare event and usually a result of abnormal anatomy or airway pathology. In elective patients, it may be predictable at the preoperative assessment (see Chapter 2).
- *Failed ventilation after intubation*: possible causes include the tube becoming kinked, blocked or disconnected, severe bronchospasm and tension pneumothorax. It may also be due to failure of the anaesthetic gas supply.
- *Aspiration*: regurgitated gastric contents can cause blockage of the airways directly or secondary to laryngeal spasm and bronchospasm. Cricoid pressure can be used to reduce the risk of regurgitation prior to intubation (see later).

Trauma

- *Directly*: during laryngoscopy and orotracheal intubation, the lips, teeth, tongue, pharynx, larynx and trachea can all be injured. In addition, during nasotracheal intubation, the nasal structures and nasopharynx can be injured. This most commonly causes bleeding and swelling.
- *Indirectly*: injury of the recurrent laryngeal nerves, and the cervical spine and cord, particularly where there is pre-existing degenerative disease or trauma.

Reflex activity

- *Hypertension and arrhythmias*: these can occur in response to laryngoscopy and intubation and may jeopardize patients, for example those with coronary artery disease or an intracranial aneurysm. In patients at risk, specific action is taken to attenuate the response – for example, pretreatment with beta-blockers or potent analgesics (fentanyl, remifentanil).
- *Vomiting*: this may be stimulated when laryngoscopy is attempted in patients who are inadequately anaesthetized. It is more frequent when there is material in the stomach, for example when the patient is not starved, in patients with intestinal obstruction or when gastric emptying is delayed, as after opiate analgesics or following trauma.
- *Laryngeal spasm*: reflex adduction of the vocal cords as a result of stimulation of the epiglottis or larynx.

Difficult and failed intubation

Occasionally it is not possible to visualize the larynx, which makes it difficult or impossible to intubate the trachea. This may have been predicted at the preoperative assessment or may be unexpected. A variety of techniques have been described to help solve this problem, which include the following.

- Manipulation of the thyroid cartilage (BURP manoeuvre) using **b**ackward, **u**pward, **r**ightward **p**ressure (patient's right) by an assistant to try and bring the larynx or its posterior aspect into view.
- At laryngoscopy, a 60 cm long gum elastic bougie is inserted blindly into the trachea, over which the tracheal tube is 'railroaded' into place.
- An LMA can be inserted and used as a conduit to pass a tracheal tube directly or via a fibreoptic bronchoscope.
- Use of indirect laryngoscopes if they are available and you have the skills necessary to use them, e.g. Glidescope®.
- Fibreoptic bronchoscopic intubation. An appropriate size and length tracheal tube is loaded onto a bronchoscope (Figure 5.8), which is then inserted via either the nose or the mouth and advanced under direct vision until it lies in the trachea. Once the bronchoscope is in the trachea, the tracheal tube is advanced off the scope until it is seen to pass the tip and also lie in the trachea. Then the bronchoscope is removed, leaving the tube in situ, the tracheal tube cuff is inflated and it is connected

to the breathing system. It is possible to perform this in a spontaneously breathing, awake, sedated patient with local anaesthesia of their airway, or after induction of general anaesthesia.

The incidence of difficult and failed intubation will depend on a number of factors, including the skill and experience of the anaesthetist and the type of cases being undertaken. A difficult or failed intubation in itself is not particularly harmful, **providing oxygenation of**

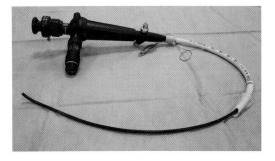

Figure 5.8 Fibreoptic intubating bronchoscope. A tracheal tube has been mounted ready to advance into the trachea.

the patient can be maintained; as most patients will have been given neuromuscular blocking drugs, they will be dependent on the anaesthetist for this. Consequently, prior to every intubation, the anaesthetic team (and surgeon if appropriate, e.g. ENT) should have devised an airway management 'strategy' and discussed this as part of the WHO surgical safety checklist. This is a series of plans that will be implemented in the event of encountering difficulty with intubation. The aim is to allow safe attempts at different methods of airway management whilst ensuring that the patient does not come to harm from hypoxia. Such plans will need to take into account the risk of aspiration and urgency of surgery, and are often referred to as plans A, B, C and D. Such a system has been developed by the Difficult Airway Society (DAS) and is outlined in Figure 5.9 [5.6]. The success or failure of each plan and the decision to move to the next plan in the strategy should be explicitly declared so that all team members are aware of what will be the next intervention. Clear communication between all anaesthetic team members is vital to a successful outcome.

Additional information including management of extubation in these patients is available on the DAS website (see Further information section).

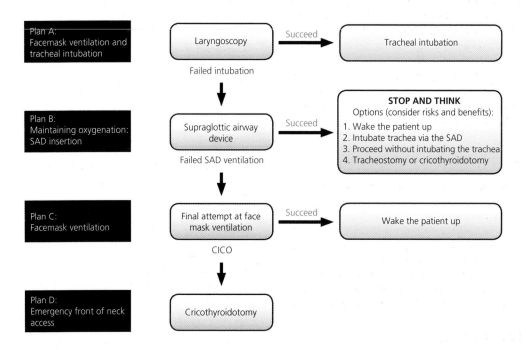

Figure 5.9 Difficult Airway Society 2015 guidelines for management of unanticipated difficult intubation in adults. Source: Frerk C, Mitchell VS, McNarry AF, *et al*. Difficult Airway Society intubation guidelines working group. *British Journal of Anaesthesia* 2015; **115**(6): 827–848. doi:10.1093/bja/aev371.

KEY POINT

- In every circumstance where difficulty is encountered with tracheal intubation, summon help immediately.

Plan A: the initial plan to use facemask ventilation followed by direct laryngoscopy to intubate the trachea. The chance of first time success should be maximized by careful attention to patient positioning, preoxygenation, muscle relaxation and choice of laryngoscope (the first choice may be a video- rather than a direct laryngoscope). Repeated attempts at laryngoscopy have the potential to cause trauma and compromise ventilation and oxygenation and view of the larynx. Therefore, a maximum of three attempts at laryngoscopy is recommended. Any repeat attempt must only be made if it is thought that something can be improved; simply repeating the same technique will have the same outcome – failure. If Plan A fails, declare a **failed intubation**.

Plan B: maintaining oxygenation. A supraglottic airway is used to ventilate the patient. If oxygenation can be maintained, then the team should 'stop and think' about what to do next. Possible options include waking the patient up, using the SGA as a conduit to attempt intubation, continuing surgery with the SGA or proceeding to a surgical airway. If ventilation or oxygenation cannot be maintained via a SGA, declare **failed SGA ventilation**.

Plan C: remove the SGA and use a facemask to oxygenate the patient. If this is successful, depending on the urgency of surgery, wake the patient up. If this fails, declare **can't intubate, can't oxygenate** (CICO).

Plan D: emergency front of neck access via cricothyroidotomy. If oxygenation is successful, a decision must be taken whether to undertake a formal tracheostomy, and whether to continue with surgery or not. In any case, the patient will need to be looked after in the critical care unit for a period.

Any patient whose airway has been traumatized, either as a result of repeated attempts at intubation or following surgical intervention, is at risk of developing oedema and airway obstruction at extubation. These patients should be admitted to an appropriate critical care area postoperatively and may require endoscopy prior to extubation. Full details of the difficulties encountered and any solutions must be documented in the patient's notes. The patient must be given verbal and written details (consider 'Medic-Alert' type device) and details sent to his or her GP. The DAS has developed an 'Airway Alert' form that contains a summary of airway management and contacts for more details (see Further information section).

Scalpel cricothyroidotomy

This involves making an incision in the front of the patient's neck, through the cricothyroid membrane, to allow a cuffed tracheal tube to be introduced. The following is a simplified description of the technique; for additional details, see the DAS website (see Further information):

- while an assistant provides rescue oxygenation via the upper airway, position the patient so that their neck is fully extended;
- standing on the patient's left-hand side (reverse if left-handed), identify the cricothyroid membrane by palpation;
- make a transverse stab incision, cutting towards you, through the skin and membrane;
- keeping the blade of the scalpel in the incision, turn it through 90°, sharp edge towards the patient's feet and apply gentle traction towards you;
- holding a bougie with your right hand, introduce it along the far side of the blade, through the incision into the trachea and advance it 10–15 cm;
- remove the scalpel and railroad a lubricated 6.0 mm cuffed tracheal tube over the bougie into the trachea;
- inflate the cuff and confirm placement with waveform capnography.

A cricothyroidotomy can be performed using a wide-bore IV cannula, alone or via a guidewire. However, this technique requires a high-pressure gas source to provide ventilation and there is a risk of barotrauma, malpositioning, kinking and blockage of the cannula. The technique should only be used by those familiar with the equipment or when the skills or facilities for performing a scalpel cricothyroidotomy are not available.

Aspiration of gastric contents

Despite a seemingly appropriate preoperative fasting period, or despite taking all of the precautions outlined above for patients identified as at risk, occasionally regurgitation and aspiration still occur [5.7]. Signs suggesting aspiration include:

- coughing during induction or recovery from anaesthesia, or during anaesthesia using a supraglottic airway device;
- gastric contents in the pharynx at laryngoscopy, or around the edge of the facemask;
- if severe, progressive hypoxia, bronchospasm and respiratory obstruction.

Occasionally, aspiration may go completely unnoticed during anaesthesia, with the development of hypoxia, hypotension and respiratory failure postoperatively.

Management
Aspiration at induction

- Maintain a patent airway and place the patient head-down and on his or her side, preferably the left; intubation is relatively easier on this side.
- Aspirate any material from the pharynx, preferably under direct vision (use a laryngoscope).

1 Neuromuscular-blocking drugs not given; surgery not urgent

- Give 100% oxygen via a facemask.
- Allow the patient to recover; give oxygen to maintain a satisfactory SpO_2.
- Treat bronchospasm with salbutamol or ipratroprium as described in Chapter 8.
- Take a chest X-ray and organize regular physiotherapy.
- Depending on degree of aspiration, consider monitoring on the ITU or high-dependency unit (HDU).

2 Neuromuscular-blocking drugs not given; surgery essential

- Get help, empty the stomach with a nasogastric tube and instil 30 mL sodium citrate.
- After allowing the patient to recover, continue using either a regional technique or a rapid-sequence induction and intubation.
- After intubation, aspirate the tracheobronchial tree and consider bronchoscopy.
- Treat bronchospasm as above.
- Postoperatively, arrange for a chest X-ray and physiotherapy.
- Recover in the ITU or HDU with oxygen therapy.
- Postoperative ventilation may be required.

3 Neuromuscular-blocking drugs given

- Intubate with a cuffed tracheal tube to secure the airway.
- Aspirate the tracheobronchial tree before starting positive pressure ventilation.
- Consider bronchopulmonary lavage with saline.
- Treat bronchospasm as above.
- Pass a nasogastric tube and empty the stomach.
- If the patient is stable (not hypoxic or hypotensive), surgery can be continued with postoperative care as described above.

If oxygen saturation remains low despite 100% oxygen, consider the possibility of obstruction and the need for fibreoptic bronchoscopy.

Aspiration intraoperatively with supraglottic airway

- Get help.
- Stop surgery if safe to do so.
- Turn patient into left lateral position with head-down tilt.
- Remove supraglottic airway device and suction oropharynx.
- Maintain ventilation with 100% oxygen and ensure ongoing anaesthesia.
- Trained assistant to apply cricoid pressure.
- Give a fast-acting neuromuscular-blocking drug and intubate the trachea.

If aspiration is suspected in a patient postoperatively, treat as for (1) above. There is no place for routine administration of large-dose steroids. Antibiotics should be given according to local protocols. In those patients with bronchospasm resistant to treatment, or with persistent hypoxia or hypotension, surgery should be deferred unless it is potentially life saving. Instead, the patient should be transferred to the ITU for ventilation, with additional, invasive cardiorespiratory monitoring as needed.

Keeping patients warm

Following the induction of anaesthesia, a forced air-warming device should be used for all patients where anaesthesia is expected to last longer than 30 minutes to prevent intraoperative hypothermia. High-risk patients (ASA II–V, preoperative temperature <36 °C, combined general and neuraxial anaesthesia, at risk of cardiovascular complications) should have forced air warming from the induction of anaesthesia, irrespective of the predicted duration. In addition, all fluids (particularly blood) should be warmed to 37 °C using a fluid warmer. Finally, inspired gases should be warmed and humidified and all non-surgical areas covered.

Maintenance of anaesthesia

The effects of the IV drug used for induction of anaesthesia will wear off after a few minutes and unconsciousness must be maintained in some other way. This can be achieved using one of a variety of inhalational anaesthetics in oxygen with or without nitrous oxide, or by an intravenous infusion of a drug (total intravenous anaesthesia – TIVA), most commonly propofol. Whether the patient breathes spontaneously or is ventilated, the principles are similar.

Inhalational anaesthesia

The patient must receive an adequate:

- concentration of oxygen to prevent hypoxia;
- concentration of anaesthetic drug to prevent awareness;
- flow of fresh gases to ensure volatile and oxygen concentrations in the breathing system remain adequate.

In order to achieve these, the composition of the gas mixture is carefully monitored. The inspired oxygen concentration is usually maintained between 30% and 50%. It is important to recognize that when a circle system is being used, this will be lower than the apparent concentration being delivered by the anaesthetic machine because of the dilutional effect of the expired gases. The anaesthetic drug used is maintained at an appropriate end-tidal concentration depending upon the patient, the surgical stimulus and the concurrent use of analgesic drugs. For the same reason, this is frequently at variance with the concentration selected on the vaporizer.

In the spontaneously breathing patient, inadequate anaesthesia for the intensity of the surgical stimulus, for example when surgery starts, will result in an increased respiratory rate and the patient may move as a result of reflex activity. In addition, there may be an increase in heart rate and blood pressure. As a result, the anaesthetist will increase the concentration of anaesthetic drug accordingly to deepen the level of unconsciousness. It may be appropriate to halt surgery temporarily while this is achieved.

In the patient who has been given neuromuscular-blocking drugs and is being ventilated, the anaesthetist must anticipate the need for changes in the depth of anaesthesia as the patient's ventilation will not change, they cannot move, and if potent opioid analgesics have been given, changes in cardiovascular signs may be minimal. Consequently, there is the possibility that the depth of anaesthesia is inadequate and the patient may be aware and unable to communicate this.

TIVA using propofol

With this technique, an appropriate brain concentration of propofol must be achieved and maintained to prevent awareness and any response to surgery. The simplest way is to give the usual IV induction dose, followed by repeated injections at intervals depending on the patient's response. This method can be used for short procedures (<10 minutes), but for maintenance over a longer period it is commoner to use a microprocessor-controlled infusion pump. This is more accurate and reliable as it uses the patient's weight and age to calculate the rate of infusion required to achieve a constant plasma (and brain) concentration. Having entered the appropriate data and started the pump, an initial rapid infusion is given to render the patient unconscious, followed by an infusion at a slower rate to maintain anaesthesia. This is often referred to as 'target-controlled infusion' (TCI). The infusion rate, and hence plasma concentration, can also be adjusted manually to take account of individual patient variation and the degree of surgical stimulation in the same way that the concentration of an inhalational anaesthetic from the vaporizer can be changed [5.8].

Propofol alone can be used to maintain anaesthesia but the infusion rates required are very high, with significant cardiovascular side-effects. It is usually combined with IV opioids, given as either repeated injections (for example, fentanyl) or an infusion (for example, remifentanil). An alternative is to use a regional anaesthetic technique for analgesia. If muscle relaxation is required, neuromuscular-blocking drugs are given and the patient is usually ventilated with oxygen-enriched air. Nitrous oxide can be used but this is not strictly TIVA and some of the advantages are lost.

 KEY POINT

- Secure venous access is essential when using TIVA.

Advantages of TIVA

- The potential toxic effects of the inhalational anaesthetics are avoided.
- The problems associated with nitrous oxide can be avoided.
- A better quality of recovery is claimed.
- It may be beneficial in certain types of surgery, for example neurosurgery.
- Pollution is reduced.

Disadvantages of TIVA

- Risk of awareness; if an IV cannula is displaced, intravenous infusion fails, or due to lack of accurate effect site anaesthetic concentration monitoring. For this reason, many would advocate depth of anaesthesia monitoring (e.g. BIS) whenever TIVA is used, especially if in conjunction with neuromuscular-blocking drugs.
- Secure, reliable intravenous access is required.
- Cost of electronic infusion pumps.
- May cause profound hypotension.

Spontaneous ventilation

Theoretically, any operation can be done with the patient breathing spontaneously. However, body cavity surgery, such as laparotomy, requires the inhibition of autonomic reflexes and significant muscle relaxation. This can only be achieved with relatively high concentrations of an inhaled or IV drug that will result in respiratory depression or even apnoea. Furthermore, at the end of surgery, as high concentrations of drugs have been given, it will take longer to excrete or eliminate them, thereby prolonging the patient's recovery. Consequently, spontaneous ventilation is used predominantly for peripheral or body surface surgery, where minimal muscle relaxation is required and autonomic reflexes can be modified by the careful titration of small doses of IV opioids or the use of regional anaesthetic techniques.

Mechanical (controlled) ventilation

The indications for using mechanical ventilation will vary amongst anaesthetists, but most would agree with using it in the following situations:

- where neuromuscular-blocking drugs are used to facilitate surgical access, for example laparotomy;
- during thoracotomy, as a negative intrathoracic pressure cannot be generated;
- when the anaesthetic technique will result in an unacceptable degree of respiratory depression;
- to allow control of carbon dioxide and thereby cerebral blood flow during neurosurgery;
- during prolonged surgical procedures;
- surgery where intubation is required, for example prone surgery, full stomach, shared airway.

The anaesthetist will have to ensure that the correct ventilator settings are used for each patient to ensure adequate alveolar ventilation while minimizing the adverse effects of positive pressure. This will require setting of:

- tidal volume and respiratory rate or;
- minute volume and tidal volume – this will then determine respiratory rate;
- the mode of ventilation (volume or pressure controlled);
- the inspiratory and expiratory times;
- peak inspiratory pressure;
- the use of positive end expiratory pressure (PEEP) if required.

Modern ventilators have a range of integral monitors and alarms that can be set to indicate if the desired ventilation is not being achieved.

The effects of positive pressure ventilation

Mechanical ventilation reverses the normal inspiratory pressure changes and has a number of important effects.

- There is an increase in the physiological dead space relative to the tidal volume and in ventilation/perfusion (V/Q) mismatch, both of which impair oxygenation. An inspired oxygen concentration of at least 30% is used to compensate for this and prevent hypoxaemia.
- The $PaCO_2$ is dependent on alveolar ventilation. Hyperventilation results in hypocapnia, causing a respiratory alkalosis. This 'shifts' the oxyhaemoglobin dissociation curve to the left, increasing the affinity of haemoglobin for oxygen. Hypocapnia will induce vasoconstriction in many organs, including the brain and heart, reducing blood flow. Underventilation will lead to hypercapnia, causing a respiratory acidosis. The effects on the oxyhaemoglobin dissociation curve are the opposite of the above, along with stimulation of the sympathetic nervous system causing vasodilatation, hypertension, tachycardia and arrhythmias.

- Excessive tidal volume may cause overdistension of the alveoli. In patients with pre-existing lung disease, this may cause a pneumothorax and, if it continues long term, a condition called ventilator-induced lung injury.
- The positive intrathoracic pressure reduces venous return to the heart and cardiac output. This effect is exaggerated in patients who are hypovolaemic.
- Both systemic and pulmonary blood flow are reduced, the latter further increasing V/Q mismatch.

Transfer into the operating theatre

At some point, the patient has to be transferred into the operating theatre. This may take place with the patient already in position and on the operating table, or they may be taken into theatre on a trolley and then transferred onto the operating table. In either case, it will often mean disconnecting the patient from the anaesthesia machine and monitoring.

Once in theatre, the first manoeuvre must be to connect the patient to the breathing circuit and ensure that they are breathing or being ventilated adequately with an appropriate gas mixture. If not already on the operating table, they are then transferred and the remaining monitoring attached. Every time a move has been completed, it is essential to ensure that the airway is not compromised and ventilation maintained. Table 5.4 shows an *aide-mémoire* to ensure patient safety.

Positioning the patient

The patient is placed in a position to facilitate surgical access and there must always be sufficient theatre staff available to achieve this task safely, both for the

patient and themselves. Some positions will require additional equipment; this must be assembled before any movement of the patient begins. The overall positioning is carried out under the direction of, and with the assistance of, the anaesthetist. At all times the prime concern remains the safety of the patient. Detailed adjustment is carried out in conjunction with the surgeon.

KEY POINT

- Every time a patient is repositioned an ABCDE check must be made to ensure safety (see Table 5.4).

The supine position (Figure 5.10)

This position is used for the majority of surgical operations, but there is no room for complacency. The patient lies flat on their back, with their head and neck in a neutral position, unless the surgeon requires otherwise, for example for surgery to the ear. The arms are placed alongside the patient's sides or flexed at the elbow lying across the lower chest. If an arm or hand is to be operated on, this limb is usually abducted and supported on an arm table. The legs are extended in a neutral position.

In this position, the abdominal contents push the diaphragm into the thorax, reducing the lung volume, in particular the functional residual capacity (FRC). There is also the tendency for dependent alveoli to be better perfused but not as well ventilated. The overall effect is to reduce oxygenation of the blood, but this can and should be compensated for by increasing the inspired oxygen concentration to a minimum of 30%.

Table 5.4 The ABCDE checklist used when moving a patient.

A: is the **A**irway, supraglottic or tracheal tube, still in place and patent?

B: are they **B**reathing, being ventilated, oxygen concentration adequate?

C: do they still have a **C**ardiac output? Monitors attached? IV drips/infusions running?

D: is the **D**epth of anaesthesia adequate? If repositioned, are all peripheral nerve protected?

E: ensure not over-**E**xposed and at risk of hypothermia

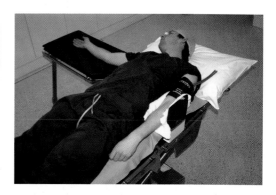
Figure 5.10 The supine position.

Points to note are as follows:

- the radial nerve is at risk from pressure midway along the humerus from a misplaced arm retainer;
- the ulnar nerve can be damaged at the elbow if allowed to lie over the edge of the mattress;
- the median nerve can be damaged in the antecubital fossa by the distal edge of the blood pressure cuff if the elbow is flexed excessively;
- the common peroneal nerve can be damaged by pressure against the head of the fibula;
- the head should be turned towards an abducted arm to reduce traction on the ipsilateral brachial plexus;
- pneumatic calf compression devices are used to reduce venous stasis in the legs and risk of deep venous thrombosis.

There are some variations in the supine position.

- *Trendelenburg*: head down, using gravity to help displace the bowels from the pelvis. Used in gynaecological and pelvic surgery.
- *Lithotomy*: with the hips and knees flexed to 90°, legs abducted slightly and the ankles supported in stirrups. Extremes of flexion and rotation must be avoided as the sciatic and femoral nerves can be damaged. The deep calf veins can be compressed against the stirrup poles. Used in gynaecological, urological and anorectal surgery.
- *Lloyd-Davies*: hips and knees flexed 30–40°, abducted and supported in gutters. This position is designed to allow the surgical team combined access to the abdomen and perineum.

The lateral position (Figure 5.11)

This is a relatively unstable position and requires a variety of additional supports to ensure the patient's safety. The anaesthetist takes responsibility for the patient's head, neck and airway and coordinates the team as the patient is turned. Depending on the site of surgery (chest, abdomen (flank) or hip), supports are placed posteriorly against the pelvis, lumbar or thoracic spine and anteriorly against the iliac crests. The upper arm is usually supported in a small gutter, again the exact position depending on site of surgery, and the lower arm is placed to lie either across the chest or adjacent to the head, flexed at the shoulder and elbow.

In this position, during mechanical ventilation, the upper lung will be preferentially ventilated while the lower lung will receive a relatively greater blood flow. This can adversely affect oxygenation, particularly in

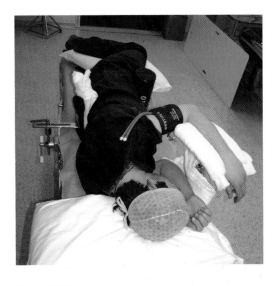

Figure 5.11 The lateral position.

patients with pre-existing pulmonary disease. More invasive monitoring may be used in this position.

There are some points to note:

- the patient's head and neck are supported to prevent traction on the brachial plexus on the uppermost side and a small support placed in the dependent axilla to prevent traction on the plexus on the patient's lower side;
- ensure that the patient's lower ear is not folded back on itself;
- take care when turning the patient to ensure that intravascular cannulas, tracheal tube and urinary catheter are not caught and removed.

The prone position (Figure 5.12)

Many variations in this position have evolved using specially designed supports. Only the basic prone position will be described here.

As described above, the anaesthetist takes control of the head and neck and coordinates the team. With arms kept at the sides, the patient is turned in two stages – firstly into the lateral position and then prone. It is essential that turning does not leave the patient flat on the table; either the head end of the table is lowered or the body raised to prevent excessive extension of the head and neck. Supports are required beneath the chest and pelvis, ensuring that the abdomen is free and the femoral vessels are not under undue pressure. The head must be supported in such a way as to prevent pressure on the eyes or tip of the nose, or occlusion of the tracheal tube. The patient's

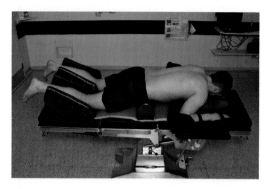

Figure 5.12 The prone position. Reproduced with permission of Dr P. Ross.

arms are either retained at the sides or flexed at the elbow and abducted at the shoulder to lie adjacent to their head. Finally, the knees are slightly flexed and padding is placed beneath the shins to raise the toes.

This position has the least detrimental effect on respiratory function. Ventilation and perfusion remain well matched, minimizing the risk of hypoxaemia. One of the main risks is obstruction of the inferior vena cava from badly placed supports reducing venous return, cardiac output and blood pressure. Careful checks must be made after turning the patient and close monitoring of the cardiovascular system is essential.

Points to note are:

- a reinforced tracheal tube is used to reduce the risk of the tube kinking – this would be difficult to correct once prone;
- great care must be taken with the cervical spine in **all** patients to prevent excessive rotation or extension;
- the arms must never be forced into position against resistance; the neck of the humerus is easily fractured;
- pressure on the eyes may cause thrombosis of the retinal artery and blindness;
- avoid compression of the femoral vessels in the groin; check the capillary refill time and colour of the feet after turning;
- ensure that pressure is not applied to the male genitalia by badly placed pelvic supports;
- avoid traction on the sciatic nerve by slightly flexing the knees;
- the abdomen must be free, particularly in spinal surgery, as compression of the inferior vena cava (IVC) will divert blood via the epidural veins that may compromise spinal surgery by excessive bleeding.

One of the commonest reasons for turning a surgical patient prone is to operate on the spine. This may be as a result of a degenerative disease processes or trauma. As the patient will have normally been given neuromuscular-blocking drugs, there will be loss of the normal muscle tone that 'protects' against excessive movement. Consequently, it is very easy to injure the spinal cord, either by placing the patient in an unsafe position or by uncontrolled or excessive movement when they are turned; the cervical spine is particularly susceptible. An experienced and fully coordinated team is essential when turning these patients.

Time out

Immediately before the start of the surgical intervention, the second stage of the WHO checklist is performed.

1 Confim that all the team members have introduced themselves by name and role.
2 The patient's identity must be confirmed, along with the planned procedure, side and site.
3 The anaesthetic, surgical and nursing teams should identify any anticipated problems, for example blood loss, equipment issues.
4 Antibiotic prophylaxis, glycaemic control and venous thromboembolism (VTE) prophylaxis have all been instituted where appropriate.
5 Imaging, for example X-rays and CT scans, is available and for the correct patient.

Once these have been confirmed and recorded, surgery can then start.

Assessment of neuromuscular blockade

This is achieved using a peripheral nerve stimulator. The electrodes can be applied to either the facial nerve, just anterior to the tragus, or over the ulnar nerve at the wrist. A variety of sequences of electrical stimulation can be used to assess the intensity of neuromuscular block. Monitoring neuromuscular block is useful during long surgical procedures, to control the timing of increments or adjust the rate of an infusion of neuromuscular-blocking drugs to prevent coughing or sudden movement. This is particularly important in some types of surgery, for example when a microscope is used as movement would be magnified and make surgery impossible, or during intracranial surgery when movement could cause significant injury to the brain from the instruments being used.

At the end of surgery, awareness of the intensity of any residual neuromuscular block allows the anaesthetist to plan reversal to ensure adequate respiratory muscle function. It can also be used when there is unexpected apnoea, to differentiate between that due to prolonged action of suxamethonium, suggesting pseudocholinesterase deficiency, and residual non-depolarizing block, when both drugs have been given. Finally, in recovery, the use of a nerve stimulator will allow the anaesthetist to distinguish between residual neuromuscular block and opioid overdose as a cause of inadequate postoperative ventilation. The former will show reduced or absent response to stimulation, the latter a normal response.

Intraoperative fluids

The type and volume of fluid given during surgery vary for each and every patient [4.4], but must take into account:

- any deficit the patient has accrued preoperatively;
- intraoperative requirements:
  - maintenance requirements during the procedure;
  - losses due to surgery;
- any vasodilatation secondary to the use of a regional anaesthetic technique (see Chapter 6).

The accrued deficit

This may be due to preoperative fasting or losses as a result of vomiting, haemorrhage or pyrexia. Any deficit due to fasting is predominantly water from the total body water volume. The volume required is calculated at the normal daily maintenance rate of 25 mL/kg/day (from the point at which fasting began). Hartmann's solution is widely used intraoperatively rather than 0.9% saline to reduce the risk of hyperchloraemic acidosis. The other main cause of a preoperative deficit is losses either from or into the gastrointestinal tract. This fluid usually contains electrolytes and effectively depletes the extracellular volume. It is best replaced with a crystalloid of similar composition, particularly in respect of the sodium concentration; for example, 0.9% sodium chloride.

Acute blood loss preoperatively can be replaced with either an appropriate volume of crystalloid (remembering that only 30% remains intravascular) or colloid. If more than 30% of the estimated blood volume has been lost (approximately 1500 mL) and bleeding is ongoing, blood should be used.

Intraoperative requirements

Maintenance fluids are usually given when surgery is prolonged (along with any accrued deficit), or if there is the possibility of a delay in the patient resuming oral fluid intake. Most patients will compensate for a preoperative deficit by increasing their oral intake postoperatively. When maintenance fluid is used, it should be given at 25 mL/kg/day, and increased if the patient is pyrexial by 10% for each degree centigrade above normal.

Losses during surgery are due to the following.

- *Evaporation*: this can occur during body cavity surgery or when large areas of tissue are exposed, depleting the total body water.
- *Trauma*: leads to the formation of tissue oedema, the volume of which is dependent upon the extent of tissue damage. This fluid is similar in composition to extracellular fluid (ECF) and is often referred to as 'third-space loss' (see Chapter 8). Third-space fluids are not of any functional use to the body, and lead to a deficit in the ECF volume.
- *Blood loss*: this will depend upon the type and site of surgery.

Fluid losses from the first two causes are difficult to measure and are extremely variable. If evaporative losses are considered excessive, then 4% glucose plus 0.18% saline can be used. Third-space losses should be replaced with a solution similar in composition to extracellular fluid, and Hartmann's is commonly used. The rate at which fluid is given and the volume required are proportional to surgical trauma and may be as much as 10 mL/kg/hour. Blood pressure, pulse, peripheral perfusion and urine output will give an indication as to the adequacy of replacement. However, in complex cases (major abdominal, urological and orthopaedic surgery), estimation of the volumes required is difficult and often inaccurate. There is now some evidence that patients whose fluid status is managed using the information provided by some form of cardiac output monitor, e.g. oesophageal Doppler or PiCCO (see Chapter 3) to monitor stroke volume and cardiac output, have better outcomes.

Blood loss is slightly more obvious and can be estimated by weighing surgical swabs and noting the volume in the suction apparatus (minus the volume of any saline washes used). Most previously well patients will tolerate the anaemia that results from the loss of 30% of their blood volume, providing that the circulating volume is adequately maintained by the use of crystalloids or colloids. Beyond this, red cell preparations are used in order to maintain the oxygen-carrying capacity of the blood. A haemoglobin level between 8 and 10 g/dL is safe even for those patients with serious cardiorespiratory disease. In most cases, the equivalent of the patient's estimated blood volume can be replaced with red cell concentrates, crystalloid and colloid in the appropriate volumes.

Occasionally, blood loss is such that the haemostatic mechanisms are affected, for example after major trauma or vascular injury. This may be seen as continuous oozing from the surgical wound or around IV cannulation sites. Most hospitals now have a 'massive transfusion protocol', which is triggered by either loss of one blood volume (estimated as 70 mL/kg) or ongoing bleeding at a rate of >150 mL/min. Blood should be taken for haemoglobin concentration, platelet count, prothrombin time (PT, or international normalized ratio – INR) and fibrinogen levels. Treatment should begin with packed cells, fresh frozen plasma and platelets, in a 1:1:1 ratio or according to local protocols. Cryoprecipitate is usually added if bleeding continues or if fibrinogen levels are low. Consideration may also be given to the use of tranexamic acid and recombinant factor VIIa.

The anaesthetic record

On every occasion an anaesthetic is given, a comprehensive and **legible** record must be made. The details and method of recording will vary with each case, the type of chart used and the equipment available. The anaesthetic record is valuable to future anaesthetists who encounter the patient, particularly when there has been a difficulty (for example, with intubation), and is also a medicolegal document, which may be referred to after several years. An anaesthetic chart typically allows the following to be recorded:

- preoperative findings, ASA grade, premedication;
- details of previous anaesthetics and any difficulties;
- apparatus used for the current anaesthetic;
- monitoring devices used;
- anaesthetic and other drugs given: timing, dose and route;
- vital signs at various intervals, usually depicted graphically;
- fluids given and lost: type and volume;
- use of local or regional anaesthetic techniques;
- anaesthetic difficulties or complications;
- postoperative instructions.

Increasingly, electronic records are being developed. These have the advantage of allowing the anaesthetist to concentrate on caring for the patient, particularly during an emergency, rather than having to stop and make a record or try to fill in the record retrospectively.

Emergence from anaesthesia

Sign out

When the surgical procedure has been completed and before any member of the team leaves the operating theatre, a number of final checks are made.

1 A final confirmation that all instruments and swabs are complete and accounted for.
2 All specimens are correctly labelled.
3 The procedure has been recorded accurately.
4 Any equipment issues that need addressing have been identified.
5 Any concerns for the immediate recovery and postoperative management for the patient are identified and recorded.

Once these have been completed, the anaesthetist has to reverse the process of anaesthesia, often referred to as 'waking the patient up'. As a consequence of the wide variety of anaesthetic techniques used, there is no absolute protocol for this stage of anaesthesia. However, there are two main priorities – recovery of consciousness and maintenance of a patent airway. Here, these will be described in relation to patients breathing spontaneously and those being ventilated.

Spontaneous ventilation, inhalational drug for maintenance, supraglottic airway

At the end of surgery, the vaporizer is turned off and the patient eliminates the inhaled anaesthetic. If a circle system is being used, the patient will continue to rebreathe the exhaled gas. This will contain some anaesthetic vapour and so the alveolar and hence plasma concentrations will only fall very slowly, delaying recovery. To speed up elimination of the anaesthetic, the flow of oxygen into the circle is increased to around 10–15 L/min. This excess flow flushes exhaled gas out of the circle, rebreathing is eliminated and the inspired oxygen concentration is almost 100%.

A supraglottic airway will now need to be removed. There are two options as to when this is done.

- Leave it in place with the patient breathing oxygen until laryngeal reflexes have been restored. The disadvantage to this is that occasionally it may result in the patient biting on the tube and obstructing the airway.
- Remove while deeply unconscious. This is easier but leaves the airway unprotected and the lack of muscle tone may result in airway obstruction and the need for the anaesthetist to perform a chin lift or jaw thrust.

Once the device has been removed, oxygen is given via a facemask and, if not already carried out, the patient is transferred from the operating table onto a trolley or bed. As the patient begins to obey commands, they can be sat up at 30° if it is safe to do so.

Mechanical ventilation, inhalational drug for maintenance, tracheal tube

The main difference from what has already been described is that normal neuromuscular function has to be restored **before** the patient regains consciousness. Therefore, recovery needs to be coordinated with the point at which the neuromuscular-blocking drug wears off spontaneously or is antagonized; this is best achieved by using a peripheral nerve stimulator. As before, the fresh gas flow is increased and the patient ventilated with 100% oxygen to eliminate the volatile drug. If necessary, a dose of neostigmine (2.5 mg) is given to antagonize the effect of the neuromuscular blocker along with an anticholinergic, usually glycopyrrolate, to block the unwanted muscarinic effects of neostigmine. Spontaneous ventilation should be restored before removal of the tracheal tube. Once ventilation commences, there are two options for when to remove the tube.

- While the patient is deeply unconscious. This leaves the airway unprotected and at risk of obstruction and the need for support by the anaesthetist or the use of an oropharyngeal airway. Furthermore, there is also the risk of the patient developing laryngospasm if any soiling of the larynx occurs as the patient recovers (for example, from saliva or regurgitated gastric contents).
- Leave in place until the patient is nearly conscious. Apart from the risk of occlusion by the patient biting the tube, the presence of the tube may also induce severe coughing and breath holding by the patient. This may cause hypoxia, as well as being painful after abdominal surgery, and undesirable after intracranial surgery as it may precipitate bleeding.

When a TIVA technique has been used to maintain anaesthesia, the principles are the same, except that the infusions are stopped to allow the plasma concentration of drug to fall to promote diffusion out of the brain. When remifentanil has been used intraoperatively, the patient will need to be given an alternative analgesic before recovering to prevent severe pain on awakening.

Anaesthetists and non-technical skills

In addition to the above, the understanding and application of non-technical skills play a major role in patient safety. Non-technical skills (also called human factors) are the cognitive, personal and social skills that complement technical skills, thereby increasing safe and efficient performance. They include team working, task management, situational awareness and decision making, all of which are underpinned by good communication skills [5.9].

The history of non-technical skills

The aviation industry, recognizing that human error was a commoner cause of aircraft accidents than equipment failure, pioneered the introduction of regular training and assessment of pilots' non-technical skills. Initially referred to as crew (or cockpit) resource management (CRM), these skills were found to contribute to improvements in aviation safety. However, until the 1990s little attention had been paid to the importance of non-technical skills in medicine and their role in medical errors. In anaesthesia, analysis of events that caused or could have caused harm to patients found that around 80% were due to problems in team working, decision making, planning and communication. As a result, Gaba and colleagues in America developed their Anesthetic Crisis Resource Management course using simulation to enhance acquisition and assessment of non-technical skills. This was followed by the Anaesthetists Non-Technical Skills (ANTS) system, pioneered by a team of anaesthetists and psychologists in Scotland. The importance of this has now spread beyond anaesthesia into many areas of healthcare [5.10].

What are non-technical skills?

Team working

A team is a group of individuals working together with a common goal; in anaesthesia this would typically be the operating theatre team. Good team members exhibit competence in their actions, are supportive to other team members, are committed to achieving the best outcome for the patient, prepared to ask for help when required and communicate well, by both listening and talking. Teams work best when they have a leader who will provide guidance to allow the team to achieve their goal. A good team leader will lead by example, relying on experience, not seniority. In addition, the team leader will know members' names, delegate wisely, be assertive when appropriate, have situational awareness (see later) and be a great communicator, empathic to all team members.

Task management

This is the planning, coordination and prioritization of the actions that are performed by the team. A good example of this in the operating theatre is the team brief before the start of the operating list, in particular planning for any untoward eventuality that may be anticipated, e.g. managing massive haemorrhage. One key feature is that team members are only allocated tasks within their areas of competence.

Situational awareness

Perhaps the easiest way of defining this skill is to rephrase it as 'knowing what is going on all around you'. This becomes particularly important when many events are happening simultaneously; this often results in a tendency to become fixated on one particular task and fail to notice something else going wrong. A good example would be during transfer of the patient from the anaesthetic room to the operating theatre: the anaesthetist concentrates on coordinating the transfer, but forgets to turn on the vaporizer on the anaesthetic machine in the operating theatre. By the time this is realized, there is a risk that the patient may have been aware. Although all team members need this skill, it must be heightened in the team leader; he or she will have to continually gather information, analyse it, plan, action and anticipate the consequences. Clearly this process is intimately linked with decision making.

Decision making

This is a process whereby an individual, usually the team leader, chooses a specific course of action from multiple alternatives available. This will require assimilation of information from all the team members along with personal observations and experience to determine the intervention. An example of this would be deciding when to perform a cricothyroidotomy in a 'can't intubate, can't oxygenate' scenario. This decision will have to be communicated clearly to all team members and once performed, the question must be asked 'did I achieve my aims?' which starts the whole cycle again.

Communication

This can be regarded as the 'glue' that holds all the other non-technical skills together. Failure of or poor communication is a constant finding when adverse events in hospitals are analysed to identify the cause. Although it is instinctive to consider words as the main form of communication, body language (or non-verbal communication) plays an important role. For communication to be effective, there are a few simple 'rules':

- direct your comments to a specific person, use their name to get their attention (or make it clear that you are addressing the whole team) and maintain eye contact while speaking to them;
- keep the information brief and to the point, concentrate on what you want to convey;
- avoid distractions, don't include unrelated facts;
- get the recipient to repeat back the important facts (sometimes known as 'call and recall');
- ask the recipient to report the results of their actions.

The aim is to create a shared mental model of the situation along with a stress-free environment.

Safety in anaesthesia is dependent on good non-technical skills. The recent development of high-fidelity simulators has facilitated the safe and effective teaching of not only technical skills, but also non-technical skills. This allows teams to repeatedly practise situations where non-technical skills are essential, particularly the management of unexpected emergencies, without any harm to patients.

FURTHER INFORMATION

Allman KG, Wilson IH (eds). *Oxford Handbook of Anaesthesia*, 4th edn. Oxford: Oxford University Press, 2016.

Cook TM, Woodall N, Frerk C. Fourth National Audit Project. Major complications of airway management in the UK: results of the Fourth National Audit Project of the Royal College of Anaesthetists. *British Journal of Anaesthesia* 2011; **106**: 266–271.

McGrath CD, Hunter JM. Monitoring of neuromuscular block. *Continuing Education in Anaesthesia, Critical Care and Pain* 2006; **6**(1): 7–12.

Spoors C, Kiff K (eds). *Training in Anaesthesia.* Oxford: Oxford University Press, 2010.

[5.1] http://anestit.unipa.it/HomePage.html
The best anaesthesia site on the web, with free sign-on. A virtual textbook of anaesthesia that includes a good section on airway management.

[5.2] http://ace.cochrane.org
This site contains systematic reviews of aspects of anaesthetic practice.

[5.3] www.aagbi.org/sites/default/files/checking_anaesthetic_equipment_2012.pdf
Checking anaesthetic equipment. AAGBI, 2012.

[5.4] www.nrls.npsa.nhs.uk/resources/?entryid45=59860
WHO safe surgery checklist adapted for use in England and Wales.

[5.5] www.nice.org.uk/guidance/ta49
Guidance from NICE on the use of ultrasound locating devices for placing central venous catheters.

[5.6] www.das.uk.com/
The Difficult Airway Society web site contains guidance on management of airway emergencies, including failed intubation drills and extubation.

[5.7] http://ceaccp.oxfordjournals.org/content/early/2013/11/21/bjaceaccp.mkt053.full
Detailed article on the risks and management of aspiration during anaesthesia and surgery.

[5.8] www.rcoa.ac.uk/salg
The Safe Anaesthesia Liaison Group, with recommendations for ensuring drug delivery during TIVA.

[5.9] www.aagbi.org/sites/default/files/anaesthesia_team_2010_0.pdf
The anaesthesia team. AAGBI, 2010.

[5.10] www.england.nhs.uk/patientsafety/
Patient safety web site with details of safety alerts, never events and reporting patient safety incidents.

6

Local and regional anaesthesia

Learning objectives

After reading this chapter you should understand the principles of:

☐ The role of local and regional anaesthesia

☐ Some of the commonly used local and regional anaesthetic techniques

☐ The advantages and disadvantages of local and regional anaesthesia

☐ How to calculate the safe dose of local anaesthetic drugs for any given patient

☐ Recognition and management of the complications of regional anaesthetic techniques

☐ Recognition and management of local anaesthetic toxicity

Apply this knowledge when practising the following skills:

☐ Calculating the maximum safe dose of local anaesthetic for a given patient

☐ Performing infiltration analgesia under supervision

When referring to local and regional techniques and the drugs used, the terms 'analgesia' and 'anaesthesia' are used loosely and interchangeably. For clarity and consistency, the following terms will be used.

- *Analgesia:* the state when only relief of pain is provided. This may allow some minor surgical procedures to be performed. An example is infiltration analgesia for suturing.
- *Anaesthesia:* the state when analgesia is accompanied by muscle relaxation, usually to allow major

surgery to be undertaken. Regional anaesthesia may be used alone or in combination with general anaesthesia.

The role of local and regional anaesthesia

The decision to use a local or regional anaesthetic technique should be based on the advantages offered to both the patient and surgeon. The following are some of the considerations taken into account:

- analgesia or anaesthesia is provided predominantly in the area required, thereby avoiding the systemic effects of drugs;

Clinical Anaesthesia: Lecture Notes, Fifth Edition. Matthew Gwinnutt and Carl Gwinnutt.
© 2017 John Wiley & Sons, Ltd. Published 2017 by John Wiley & Sons, Ltd.
Companion website: www.lecturenoteseries.com/anaesthesia

- spontaneous ventilation is preserved and respiratory depressant drugs can be avoided in patients with chronic respiratory disease;
- there is generally less disturbance of the control of co-existing systemic disease requiring medical therapy, such as diabetes mellitus;
- the airway reflexes are preserved and, in a patient with a full stomach, particularly due to delayed gastric emptying (for example, in pregnancy), the risk of aspiration is reduced;
- central neural blockade may improve access and facilitate surgery, for example by causing contraction of the bowel or by providing profound muscle relaxation;
- blood loss can be reduced with controlled hypotension;
- there is a considerable reduction in the equipment required and the cost of anaesthesia – this may be important in underdeveloped areas;
- when used in conjunction with general anaesthesia, only sufficient anaesthetic (inhalational or intravenous (IV)) is required to maintain unconsciousness, with analgesia and muscle relaxation provided by the regional technique;
- some techniques can be continued postoperatively to provide pain relief, for example an epidural;
- complications after major surgery are significantly reduced, e.g. respiratory failure after upper abdominal or thoracic surgery.

 KEY POINT

- Regional anaesthesia is not just an answer to the problem of anaesthesia in patients regarded as not well enough for general anaesthesia.

General considerations

Any regional or local anaesthetic technique should be discussed with the patient beforehand and an explanation given of the procedure to be performed, the risks, benefits and any alternatives, if appropriate, to allow informed consent to be obtained. Increasingly, written consent is being obtained. Initial objections and fears are best alleviated and usually overcome by explanation of the advantages and by reassurance. A patient should never be forced to accept a local or regional technique.

In all patients in whom regional or local anaesthesia is planned, enquire specifically about whether the patient is taking any anticoagulant or antiplatelet medications and if indicated, check recent coagulation results and platelet count [6.1].

An understanding of the surgery planned and the nerve supply of the area to be operated on is necessary in order to select the appropriate regional technique. For example, if a regional anaesthetic technique alone is planned and a limb tourniquet is to be used, the location of the tourniquet must also be adequately anaesthetized. Additional analgesia should be planned to start in advance of when the regional block is anticipated to wear off so that the patient is not left in pain at this point.

Whenever a local or regional anaesthetic technique is used, facilities for resuscitation and for converting to a general anaesthetic must always be available immediately in order that allergic reactions, toxicity, failure or inadequate anaesthesia can be dealt with effectively. As a minimum this will include the following:

- equipment to maintain and secure the airway, give oxygen and provide ventilation;
- intravenous cannulas and a range of fluids;
- drugs, including adrenaline, atropine, vasopressors and anticonvulsants;
- suction.

Patients should always be on a trolley or operating table that is capable of being tipped head down.

Local and regional anaesthetic techniques

Local anaesthetic drugs can be used:

- topically on a mucous membrane, such as the eye or urethra;
- for subcutaneous infiltration;
- directly around nerves, for example the brachial plexus;
- in the extradural space ('epidural anaesthesia');
- in the subarachnoid space ('spinal anaesthesia').

The latter two techniques are more correctly called 'central neuraxial blockade'; however, the term 'spinal anaesthesia' is commonly used when local anaesthetic is injected into the subarachnoid space and it is in this context that it will be used here.

The following is a brief introduction to some of the more popular regional anaesthetic techniques; further details can be found on the Regional Anaesthesia UK (RAUK) website [6.2]. Recently, there has been increased awareness of local anaesthetic blocks being performed on the wrong side. This has resulted in guidelines being produced to reduce this risk [6.3].

Infiltration analgesia

Lidocaine 1–2% is used for short procedures, for example suturing a wound, and 0.2–0.5% bupivacaine or levo-bupivacaine for pain relief from a surgical incision. A solution containing adrenaline can be used if a large dose or a prolonged effect is required, providing that tissues around end arteries are avoided. Infiltration analgesia is not instantaneous and lack of patience is the commonest reason for failure. The technique used is as follows.

1. Calculate the maximum volume of drug that can be used (see Chapter 4).
2. Clean the skin surrounding the wound with an appropriate solution and allow it to dry.
3. Insert the needle subcutaneously, avoiding any obvious blood vessels.
4. Aspirate to ensure that the tip of the needle does not lie in a blood vessel. If blood is aspirated, discard the syringe and start again.
5. Inject the local anaesthetic in a constant flow as the needle is withdrawn. Too rapid injection will cause pain.
6. Second and subsequent punctures should be made through an area of skin already anaesthetized.
7. In a clean wound, local anaesthetic can be injected directly into the exposed wound edge. This technique can also be used at the end of surgery to help reduce wound pain postoperatively.

Brachial plexus block

The nerves of the brachial plexus can be anaesthetized by injecting the local anaesthetic drug either above the level of the clavicle (supraclavicular approach or interscalene approach) or where the nerves enter the arm through the axilla along with the axillary artery and vein (axillary approach). Ultrasound guidance with or without a nerve stimulator is used to visualize needle insertion and deposition of local anaesthetic, thereby increasing the effectiveness of the 'block' whilst avoiding nerve injury and intravascular injection of the local anaesthetic drug. All of the drugs in Table 4.10 can be used. These techniques can be used for a wide range of surgical procedures; interscalene blocks are used for shoulder surgery whereas an axillary block is useful for operations below the elbow. Both will provide good analgesia in the immediate postoperative period. The block may last several

hours, and so it is important to warn both the surgeon and patient of this.

Transversus abdominis plane (TAP) block

As the name suggests, this block aims to deposit local anaesthetic in the plane between the transversus abdominis and internal oblique muscles (Figure 6.1a) to anaesthetize the nerves supplying the skin and muscles of the anterior abdominal wall (and parietal peritoneum). Ultrasound guidance is used to locate the correct plane between the muscles.

The needle is inserted in the midaxillary line midway between the costal margin and iliac crest. When

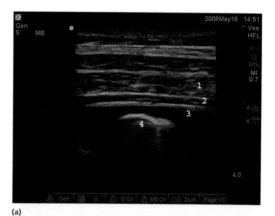
(a)

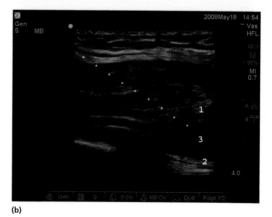
(b)

Figure 6.1 (a) Ultrasound image of anatomy for TAP block. (1) Internal oblique, (2) transversus abdominis, (3) peritoneal cavity, (4) bowel. (b) Ultrasound image of TAP block. (1) Internal oblique, (2) displaced transversus abdominis, (3) pool of local anaesthetic solution. Dotted line indicates position of needle. Source: courtesy of Dr J. Corcoran.

the needle reaches the correct plane, 2–3 mL saline is injected to confirm the location, followed by the local anaesthetic (Figure 6.1b). Alternatively, a catheter can be inserted and an infusion of local anaesthetic given for prolonged analgesia. For midline incisions, bilateral blocks will be required and care must be taken not to exceed the maximum safe dose of local anaesthetic. The block is most useful in lower abdominal surgery, for example appendicectomy, hernia repair, abdominal hysterectomy and laparoscopic surgery.

Epidural anaesthesia

Epidural (extradural) anaesthesia involves the deposition of a local anaesthetic drug into the potential space **outside** the dura (Figure 6.2a). This space extends from the craniocervical junction at C1 to the sacrococcygeal membrane, and anaesthesia can theoretically be safely instituted at any level in between. In practice, an epidural is sited adjacent to the nerve roots that supply the surgical site; that is, the lumbar region is used for pelvic and lower limb surgery and

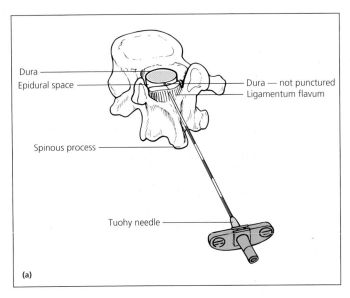

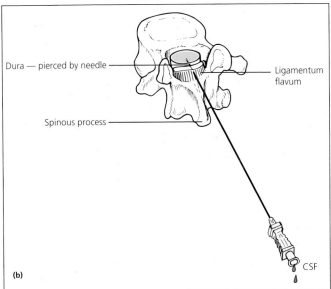

Figure 6.2 (a) Placement of the needle tip for epidural anaesthesia. (b) Placement of the needle tip for spinal (intrathecal) anaesthesia. Source: Gwinnutt CL. *Clinical Anaesthesia*. Oxford: Blackwell Science, 1996.

the thoracic region for abdominal surgery. A single injection of local anaesthetic can be given but more commonly, a catheter is inserted into the epidural space and either repeated injections or a constant infusion of a local anaesthetic drug is used.

To aid identification of the epidural space, a technique termed 'loss of resistance' is used. The (Tuohy) needle is advanced until its tip is embedded within the ligamentum flavum (yellow ligament). This blocks the tip and causes marked resistance to attempted injection of saline or air from a syringe attached to the needle. As the needle is advanced further, the ligament is pierced, resistance disappears dramatically and saline/air is injected easily. The needle has markings every 1 cm to enable determination of the depth of the epidural space.

A plastic catheter is then inserted into the epidural space via the needle. The catheter is marked at 5 cm intervals to 20 cm with extra markings every 1 cm between 5 and 15 cm. Knowing how far the catheter has been inserted, as well as the depth of the epidural space, allows calculation of the length of the catheter in the epidural space.

Varying concentrations of local anaesthetics can be used depending on the effect desired. When using bupivacaine or levo-bupivacaine, 0.5% will be needed for surgical anaesthesia with muscle relaxation, but only 0.1–0.2% for postoperative analgesia. Local anaesthetic will spread from the level of injection both up and down the epidural space. The extent of anaesthesia is determined by:

- the spinal level of insertion of the epidural: for a given volume, spread is greater in the thoracic region than in the lumbar region;
- the volume of local anaesthetic injected;
- gravity: tipping the patient head down encourages spread cranially, while head up tends to limit spread.

The spread of anaesthesia is described with reference to the limits of the dermatomes affected; for example, the inguinal ligament, T12; the umbilicus, T10; and the nipples, T4. An opioid is often given with the local anaesthetic to improve the quality and duration of analgesia, for instance fentanyl or diamorphine. For details of infusions of local anaesthetics and opioids for postoperative analgesia, see Chapter 7.

Spinal anaesthesia

Spinal anaesthesia results from the injection of a local anaesthetic drug directly into the cerebrospinal fluid (CSF) within the subarachnoid (intrathecal) space

(Figure 6.2b). The spinal needle can only be inserted below the second lumbar and above the first sacral vertebra; the upper limit is determined by the termination of the spinal cord and the lower limit because the sacral vertebrae are fused and access becomes virtually impossible. When the tip of the needle is correctly positioned, CSF will appear at the hub (Figure 6.3). A single injection of local anaesthetic is normally used, thereby limiting the duration of the technique.

A fine, 24–29 G needle with a 'pencil point' or tapered point (for example, a Whitacre or Sprotte needle) is used (Figure 6.4). The small diameter and shape are an attempt to reduce the incidence of postdural puncture headache (see later). To aid passage of this needle

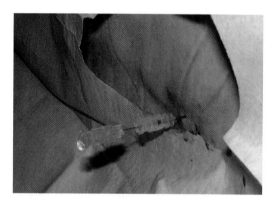

Figure 6.3 Spinal anaesthesia. The 25 G needle has been inserted via an introducer and CSF can be seen dripping from the hub.

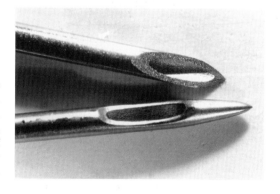

Figure 6.4 Photomicrograph showing the shape of a bevel needle (*top*) and 'pencil point' needle (*below*). Source: Jones MJ, Selby IR, Gwinnutt CL and Hughes DG. Technical note: the influence of using an atraumatic needle on the incidence of post-myelography headache. *British Journal of Radiology* 1994; 67: 396–398.

through the skin and interspinous ligament, a short, wide-bore 'introducer' needle is inserted initially and the spinal needle is passed through its lumen.

Factors influencing the spread of the local anaesthetic drug within the CSF, and hence the extent of anaesthesia, include the following.

- The specific gravity (baricity) of the anaesthetic solution relative to CSF. Hyperbaric (heavy) solutions, for example 'heavy' bupivacaine (0.5%), will sink within the CSF and upward spread will be limited and can be controlled by positioning the patient. Hyperbaricity is achieved by the addition of 8% dextrose.
- Positioning of the patient either during or after the injection. Maintenance of the sitting position after injection results in a block of the low lumbar and sacral nerves. In the supine position, the block will extend to the thoracic nerves around T5–6, the point of maximum backwards curve (kyphosis) of the thoracic spine. Further extension can be obtained with a head-down tilt.
- Increasing the dose (volume and/or concentration) of local anaesthetic drug.
- The higher the placement of the spinal anaesthetic in the lumbar region, the higher the level of block obtained.

Small doses of an opioid, for example fentanyl 12.5–50 µg or diamorphine 250–500 µg, may be injected with the local anaesthetic. This extends the duration of analgesia for up to 12 hours postoperatively.

Contraindications to epidural and spinal anaesthesia

- *Hypovolaemia:* as a result of either blood loss or dehydration. Such patients are likely to experience severe falls in cardiac output as any compensatory vasoconstriction is lost.
- *A low, fixed cardiac output:* as seen with severe aortic or mitral stenosis. The reduced venous return further reduces cardiac output, jeopardizing perfusion of vital organs.
- *Local skin sepsis:* risk of introducing infection.
- *Coagulopathy:* as a result of either a bleeding diathesis (for example, haemophilia) or therapeutic anticoagulation. This risks causing an epidural haematoma. There may also be a very small risk in patients taking aspirin and associated drugs that reduce platelet activity. Where heparins are used perioperatively to reduce the risk of deep venous thrombosis, these may be started after the insertion of the epidural or spinal.

- *Raised intracranial pressure:* a risk of precipitating coning.
- *Known allergy to amide local anaesthetic drugs.*
- *A patient who is totally uncooperative.*
- *Concurrent disease of the central nervous system (CNS):* some would caution against the use of these techniques for fear of being blamed for any subsequent deterioration.
- *Previous spinal surgery or abnormal spinal anatomy:* although not an absolute contraindication, epidural or spinal anaesthesia may be technically difficult.

Monitoring during local and regional anaesthesia

During epidural and spinal anaesthesia, the guidelines on monitoring (see Chapter 5) should be followed. Particular attention must be paid to the cardiovascular system as a result of the profound effects these techniques can have. Maintenance of verbal contact with the patient is useful as it gives an indication of cerebral perfusion. Early signs of inadequate cardiac output are complaints of nausea and faintness, and subsequent vomiting. The first indication of extensive spread of anaesthesia may be a complaint of difficulty with breathing or numbness in the fingers. When epidural or spinal anaesthesia is used, patients are often also sedated (e.g. with midazolam), but this must be carefully titrated as valuable signs and symptoms will be lost, and airway reflexes and ventilation impaired if the patient is too heavily sedated.

 KEY POINT

- A conscious patient is not an excuse for inadequate monitoring.

Complications of central neural blockade

These are usually mild and rarely cause any lasting morbidity (Table 6.1). Those commonly seen intraoperatively are predominantly due to the effects of the

Table 6.1 Incidence of common complications with spinal anaesthesia.

• Hypotension	33%
• Nausea	18%
• Bradycardia	13%
• Vomiting	7%
• Dysrhythmias	2%
• Postdural puncture headache	<1%

local anaesthetic [6.4]. Their management is covered later in this chapter. Complications seen in patients receiving epidural analgesia postoperatively are covered in Chapter 8.

Hypotension and bradycardia

Anaesthesia of the lumbar and thoracic nerves results in progressive sympathetic block causing vasodilatation, a reduction in the peripheral resistance and venous return to the heart, and a fall in cardiac output. If the block extends cranially beyond T5, the cardioaccelerator nerves are also blocked, and unopposed vagal tone results in a bradycardia. Small falls in blood pressure are tolerated and may be helpful in reducing blood loss. If the blood pressure falls by >25% of resting value, or the patient becomes symptomatic (see later), treatment consists of:

- oxygen via a facemask;
- IV fluids (crystalloids or colloids) to increase venous return;
- vasopressors to counteract the vasodilatation, either ephedrine, an alpha- and beta-agonist (3 mg IV) or metaraminol, an alpha-agonist (0.25 mg IV);
- atropine 0.3–0.6 mg IV if a bradycardia causes haemodynamic compromise.

Nausea and vomiting

These are most often the first indications of hypotension and cerebral hypoperfusion but can also result from vagal stimulation during upper abdominal surgery. Any hypotension or hypoxia is corrected as described earlier. If due to surgery, try to reduce the degree of manipulation. If this is not possible then it may be necessary to convert to general anaesthesia. Atropine 0.3–0.6 mg IV is frequently effective, particularly if there is a bradycardia. Antiemetics can

be tried (for example, ondansetron 4 mg IV), but this must not be at the expense of the above.

Postdural puncture headache (PDPH)

This is caused by a persistent leak of CSF from the needle hole in the dura. The incidence is greatest with large holes, most commonly due to inadvertent dural puncture with a Tuohy during epidural anaesthesia, and least after spinal anaesthesia using fine needles (for example, 26 G) and with a pencil or tapered point (<1%). Patients usually complain of a headache that is frontal or occipital, postural and exacerbated by straining. The majority will resolve spontaneously. Persistent headaches can normally be relieved (in >90% cases) by injecting 20–30 mL of the patient's own venous blood into the epidural space (epidural blood patch) under strict aseptic conditions.

Local anaesthetic toxicity

This is usually the result of one of the following.

- *Rapid absorption of a normally safe dose:* use of an excessively concentrated solution or injection into a vascular area results in rapid absorption.
- *Inadvertent IV injection:* failure to aspirate prior to injection via virtually any route.
- *Overdose:* failure or error in either calculating the maximum safe dose or taking into account any pre-existing cardiac or hepatic disease.

Signs and symptoms of toxicity are due to effects on the CNS and the cardiovascular system. These are dependent on the plasma concentration and initially may represent either a mild toxicity or, more significantly, the early stages of a more severe reaction.

- *Mild or early:* circumoral paraesthesia, numbness of the tongue, visual disturbances, light-headedness, slurred speech, twitching, restlessness, mild hypotension and bradycardia.
- *Severe or late:* grand mal convulsions followed by coma, respiratory depression and eventually apnoea, cardiovascular collapse with profound hypotension and bradycardia, and ultimately cardiac arrest.

The incidence of severe systemic toxicity varies from 1 in 1000 with peripheral nerve blocks to 1 in 10 000 with epidural anaesthesia

Management of toxicity

If a patient complains of any of the above symptoms or exhibits signs, stop giving the local anaesthetic immediately! The next steps are as follows.

- *Get help:* several actions will need to be performed simultaneously, especially if the toxicity is severe.
- *Airway:* maintain using basic techniques. Tracheal intubation will be needed if the protective reflexes are absent to protect against aspiration.
- *Breathing:* give oxygen (100%) with support of ventilation if inadequate.
- *Circulation:* raise the patient's legs to encourage venous return and start an IV infusion of crystalloid or colloid. Treat a bradycardia with IV atropine.
- *Disability:* convulsions must be treated early. Diazepam 5–10 mg intravenously can be used initially but this may cause significant respiratory depression. If the convulsions do not respond or they recur, then seek expert advice.

Circulatory collapse

If local anaesthetic toxicity causes profound circulatory collapse and cardiac arrest, intravenous lipid emulsion should be given [6.5]. The aim of this is to bind the local anaesthetic molecules in the plasma and reduce the amount that is free to bind to cardiac tissue. In such circumstances, the AAGBI has issued the following guidelines [6.6]:

- in cardiac arrest, start cardiopulmonary resuscitation (CPR) using current guidelines;
- manage any arrhythmias according to current protocols (don't use lidocaine as an antiarrhythmic!);
- start IV lipid emulsion therapy:
  - give 1.5 mL/kg 20% lipid emulsion (approximately 100 mL) over 1 minute;
  - start an infusion of 20% lipid emulsion at a rate of 15 mL/kg/h;
- after 5 minutes, if cardiovascular stability has not been restored or an adequate circulation deteriorates:
  - repeat two further boluses, 5 minutes apart;
  - double the rate of the infusion;
- do not exceed a maximum dose of 12 mL/kg.

If resuscitation is ongoing or successful, the patient should be transferred to a critical care area. The patient should be monitored for at least 48 hours for the development of pancreatitis (a potential complication of lipid emulsion therapy) and the case should be reported to the National Patient Safety Agency (NPSA) in the UK and can be reported to www.lipidrescue.org.

Because of the risk of an inadvertent overdose of a local anaesthetic drug, they should only be given where full facilities for monitoring and resuscitation are immediately available. This ensures the maximum chance of patient recovery without any permanent sequelae.

Regional anaesthesia: in awake or anaesthetized patients?

Major nerve blocks and epidural anaesthesia are often combined with general anaesthesia to reduce the amount and number of systemic drugs given, and to provide postoperative analgesia. Claimed advantages of performing the block with the patient awake are:

- the block can be checked before surgery commences to ensure it works satisfactorily;
- the risk of nerve injury is reduced as the patient will complain if the needle touches a nerve;
- the patient can cooperate with positioning.

Advantages claimed for performing the block after induction of anaesthesia are:

- it is more pleasant for the patient, with no discomfort during insertion of the needle;
- there is no risk of the patient moving suddenly;
- it allows easier positioning of patients in pain, for example due to fractures;
- if the needle hits the nerve then the damage has already been done.

Fortunately, in experienced hands with either technique, the risk of nerve injury resulting in permanent sequelae is very rare. However, all patients who have a regional technique should be assessed to ensure that there is full recovery of normal function.

FURTHER INFORMATION

Fischer HBJ, Pinnock CA (eds). *Fundamentals of Regional Anaesthesia*. Cambridge: Cambridge University Press, 2004.

Nicholls B, Conn D, Roberts A. *The Abbott Pocket Guide to Practical Peripheral Nerve Blockade*. Maidenhead: Abbott Anaesthesia, 2008.

Spoors C, Kiff K (eds). *Training in Anaesthesia*. Oxford: Oxford University Press, 2010.

[6.1] www.aagbi.org/sites/default/files/rapac_2013_web.pdf
Recent guidelines on regional anaesthesia in patients with abnormalities or coagulation.

[6.2] www.youtube.com/user/RAUKvideos
Useful video clips of blocks being performed under ultrasound from Regional Anaesthesia United Kingdom (RAUK).

[6.3] http://salg.ac.uk/standards-of-clinical-practice/wrong-site-block
Toolkit from the Royal College of Anaesthetists, Safe Anaesthesia Liaison Group and the Safety Network aimed at reducing the risks from local anaesthetic blocks.

[6.4] www.rcoa.ac.uk/nap3
The report of National Audit Project 3 looking into the complications of neuraxial block in the UK, 2009. Executive summary and full report.

[6.5] www.lipidrescue.squarespace.com
Site dedicated to improving knowledge on the use of lipid to treat cardiac toxicity following local anaesthetic overdose.

[6.6] www.aagbi.org/sites/default/files/la_toxicity_2010_0.pdf
Downloadable chart for management of severe local anaesthetic toxicity.

7

Specialized areas of anaesthesia

Learning objectives

After reading this chapter you should understand the principles of anaesthesia for:

☐ Emergency surgery

☐ Obstetrics

☐ Thoracic surgery

☐ The overweight and obese

☐ Children

Apply this knowledge when practising the following skills:

☐ Applying cricoid pressure during induction of anaesthesia and tracheal intubation

☐ Positioning a patient undergoing caesarean section to prevent aortocaval compression

☐ Calculating the dose of drugs for an obese patient

☐ Calculating the weight of a child knowing its age

The principles underlying anaesthesia have been covered in earlier chapters. However, there are a number of anaesthetic subspecialties which have significant differences in practice and they merit a brief introduction. This chapter covers the key areas, recognizing that there are others.

Anaesthesia for emergency surgery

Being able to anaesthetize safely those who require emergency surgery is an essential skill for all anaesthetists [7.1]. The following is an outline of the key issues.

Clinical Anaesthesia: Lecture Notes, Fifth Edition. Matthew Gwinnutt and Carl Gwinnutt.
© 2017 John Wiley & Sons, Ltd. Published 2017 by John Wiley & Sons, Ltd.
Companion website: www.lecturenoteseries.com/anaesthesia

It is assumed that patients who need anaesthetizing for emergency surgery will not have an empty stomach, which poses an increased risk of regurgitation and aspiration into the lungs of acidic stomach contents. The greatest risk is during induction of anaesthesia but some patients are also at risk during extubation and recovery. The incidence of complications appears to be related to both the volume (>25 mL) and pH (<2.5) of the material aspirated. Factors predisposing to aspiration include the following.

- *A full stomach*: an inadequate period of starvation (emergency patients), increased gastrointestinal contents secondary to bowel obstruction, distension following facemask ventilation.
- *Delayed gastric emptying*: drugs (especially opiates), trauma (particularly head injury),

peritoneal irritation, blood in the stomach, pain and anxiety.

- *Obstetric patients* (see later in this chapter).
- *Other causes*: a history of gastro-oesophageal reflux, hiatus hernia, obesity, head-down position, presence of a bulbar palsy, oesophageal pouch or stricture.

Consequently, in these patients, measures will be taken to prevent aspiration and the majority will be intubated in order to secure and protect their airway. In order to achieve this as safely as possible, the technique used for induction of anaesthesia is slightly modified and referred to as rapid-sequence induction or RSI.

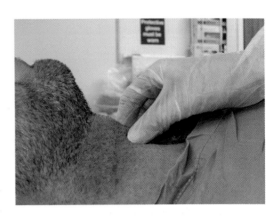

Figure 7.1 Cricoid pressure (Sellick's manoeuvre).

Reducing the risks of aspiration

A variety of methods are used, alone or in combination.

1 Reduction of residual gastric volume:
- an adequate period of preoperative starvation;
- avoidance of drugs that delay gastric emptying;
- insertion of a nasogastric tube and aspiration of gastric contents;
- use of prokinetic drugs, such as metoclopramide.

2 Increase pH of gastric contents:
- sodium citrate to neutralize gastric acid;
- H1 antagonists, e.g. oral or intravenous (IV) rantidine (whichever route is most appropriate);
- proton pump inhibitors (PPIs), for example omeprazole, lansoprazole (conveniently available in an oro-dispersible preparation).

3 Use of cricoid pressure (see later).

Cricoid pressure (Sellick's manoeuvre)

Aspiration of regurgitated gastric contents is a life-threatening complication of anaesthesia and every effort must be made to minimize the risk. Cricoid pressure is used as a physical barrier to regurgitation in patients at high risk of regurgitation. The cricoid cartilage is the only complete ring of cartilage in the larynx. Pressure applied to its anterior aspect forces the whole ring posteriorly, compressing the oesophagus against the body of the sixth cervical vertebra, occluding it and preventing regurgitation. The manoeuvre is carried out by an assistant, applying pressure as the patient loses consciousness, using the thumb and index finger of their right hand whilst the other hand stabilizes the patient's neck from behind (Figure 7.1). Cricoid pressure should be maintained even if the patient starts to actively vomit, as the risk of aspiration is greater than the theoretical risk of oesophageal rupture.

Rapid-sequence induction of anaesthesia

Preoxygenation is achieved (see Chapter 5), during which time monitors are attached, venous access is secured if not already done and an intravenous (IV) infusion started. Suction apparatus is switched on and a rigid Yankauer sucker attached and placed within immediate reach of the anaesthetist. A check is made that the anaesthetic assistant is able to apply cricoid pressure effectively and they understand it is not to be released until instruction is given by the anaesthetist to do so. Patients must also be warned that they will feel gentle pressure on their neck.

When preoxygenation is judged to be adequate, gentle cricoid pressure (10 N) is applied and the predetermined dose of the induction drug is given into a fast-running IV infusion and, as consciousness is lost, the cricoid pressure is increased (30 N). The dose of suxamethonium is given and the facemask is held against the patient's face, but manual ventilation is not performed. To do so would risk forcing oxygen into the stomach, distending it and increasing the risk of regurgitation. The patient is observed for the fasciculations caused by suxamethonium and once they have stopped, direct laryngoscopy is performed and the patient intubated. The cuff of the tracheal tube is inflated and satisfactory position of the tube confirmed as already described. When the anaesthetist is confident that the tube is in the trachea, cricoid pressure is released.

Anaesthesia and surgery then continue as described previously, using either an inhalational or intravenous technique to maintain anaesthesia. A non-depolarizing neuromuscular-blocking drug is given when there is evidence, either clinically or by using a nerve stimulator, that the effect of suxamethonium is diminishing. It is common to pass a nasogastric (or orogastric) tube during anaesthesia to allow aspiration of gastric contents. However, this does not always guarantee complete emptying of the stomach. Therefore, at the end of surgery, patients are extubated once there is evidence of return of their laryngeal reflexes (for example, coughing), with them sat up at 30° or, if this is not appropriate, on their side.

Anaesthesia for obstetric patients

Obstetric patients may require anaesthesia for a variety of surgical procedures but the commonest is for a caesarean section, either electively or as an emergency, usually when the mother is already in labour. The following is an outline of the principles of anaesthesia [7.2]. It is important to note that, whichever technique is used, adequate prophylaxis against acid aspiration is mandatory.

- Elective caesarean section – an H1 antagonist or proton pump inhibitor the night before and morning of surgery.
- Emergency caesarean section – an H1 antagonist and 30 mL 0.3 M sodium citrate immediately before going to theatre.

There are two main anaesthetic techniques for a caesarean section: regional (epidural or spinal anaesthesia) and general anaesthesia. Current recommendations are that caesarean section should wherever possible be performed under regional anaesthesia as this is associated with lower maternal and foetal mortality [7.3].

Regional anaesthesia is now the choice for almost all elective (90%) and most emergency caesarean sections, and the majority of these are spinal anaesthetics as this provides rapid, reliable and intense anaesthesia. It is recommended that women are offered intrathecal diamorphine as part of the technique, as this improves postoperative pain control and reduces the need for further analgesia.

The principles of spinal anaesthesia are as described in Chapter 5. Most anaesthetists perform the spinal with the patient sitting as this makes the midline easier to identify and is associated with slightly faster onset of block. The main problems associated with this technique are that unlike general and epidural anaesthesia, it is time limited and hypotension is commoner. The latter is usually managed with a combination of an IV fluid preload and an infusion of phenylephrine (30–60 µg/minute).

Epidurals are predominantly used to provide analgesia during labour. The extent and intensity of the block can be increased (anaesthesia) to allow caesarean section to take place. However, this is a relatively slow process and there is a risk of inadequate anaesthesia due to inadequate or absent block of some nerve roots. The technique and other problems are as described in Chapter 5.

The commonest reasons for the use of general anaesthesia are the urgency of the caesarean section (usually because of an immediate threat to the life of the mother or foetus), refusal of a regional technique by the patient, failure or contraindication of the regional technique. There are a number of problems specifically associated with general anaesthesia.

- There is an increased risk of regurgitation and aspiration. This is due to the progesterone-induced relaxation of the lower oesophageal sphincter and increased intra-abdominal pressure from the presence of the gravid uterus. This is exacerbated by the fact that in labour, gastric emptying is very slow. All pregnant women requiring general anaesthesia are regarded as having a full stomach and receive antacid prophylaxis as described above and anaesthesia is induced using an RSI with cricoid pressure. During emergency surgery, a gastric tube is passed to try and empty the stomach, and patients should be extubated once there is evidence of return of their laryngeal reflexes (e.g. coughing) and sat up at 30°.
- Failed intubation is commoner in obstetric patients (1:300 compared to 1:3000 non-obstetric patients). This is primarily due to anatomical factors, in particular enlargement of breast tissue, engorgement of the airway mucosa and the fact that most women have a full set of teeth. When combined with the fact that the functional residual capacity (FRC) is reduced and oxygen consumption increased, the pregnant woman will desaturate and become hypoxic remarkably quickly during repeated attempts at intubation. Attention must be paid to ensuring full preoxygenation, head and neck position must be optimized, and

intubation must only be attempted at the point of maximal action of suxamethonium. If intubation fails, institute a failed intubation drill. Oxygenation is more important than intubation.

- Maternal awareness as a result of the use of inadequate doses of the induction and inhalational drugs in an attempt to avoid oversedating the baby. Adequate doses of drugs must be given; 'flat' babies can be resuscitated by a paediatrician.

Aortocaval compression

As the gravid uterus enlarges through the pregnancy, it compresses the inferior vena cava, reducing venous return to the heart and therefore cardiac output and blood pressure. The effect is maximal by 36 weeks gestation, worse in the supine position and exacerbated by the sympathetic block produced by epidurals and spinals. In addition, compression of the aorta may occur, reducing blood pressure and flow in the uterine arteries that may cause foetal hypoxia. Both of these effects can be prevented by using a 15° left lateral tilt in the supine patient and it is essential that, whichever technique of anaesthesia is used for a caesarean section, the mother is placed in this position (Figure 7.2).

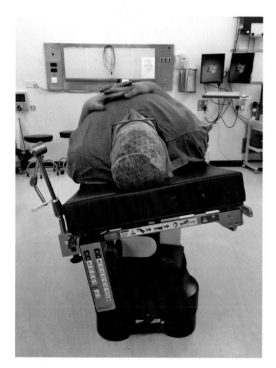

Figure 7.2 Patient (volunteer) positioned on operating table with 15° left lateral tilt.

 KEY POINT

- All women undergoing caesarean section must be positioned with 15° left lateral tilt to prevent aortocaval compression.

Anaesthesia for thoracic surgery

Surgery to the chest contents or to the anterior thoracic spine via a thoracotomy poses significant challenges for the anaesthetist – in particular the need to isolate and ventilate both lungs independently. This allows one lung to be deflated whilst ventilation is maintained via the other. The indications for this are to:

- facilitate surgical access, for example to the oesophagus, thoracic spine, the deflated lung;
- avoid contamination from one lung to the other, for example infection, bleeding;
- allow differential ventilation of both lungs, for example in the presence of a large leak due to a bronchopleural fistula.

The most popular method of achieving one-lung ventilation (OLV) is by the insertion of a double-lumen tube (Figure 7.3). A variety of suitable tubes are available, made out of either natural 'red' rubber or PVC (single use). The principle of these tubes is that one lumen is longer and designed to be introduced specifically into the left or right main bronchus (hence they are referred to as left- or right-sided endobronchial tubes). A small cuff on this bronchial lumen provides a gas-tight seal and allows ventilation of the lung on this side. The other, shorter lumen ends proximal to the carina, has a larger cuff and gas delivered down this lumen predominantly enters the non-intubated bronchus. These tubes are considerably larger than standard tracheal tubes and can be difficult to insert to lie in the correct position. Therefore, after insertion, their position is checked clinically by checking that both lungs can be ventilated independently, and many anaesthetists will confirm placement by inserting a bronchoscope [7.4].

After insertion, both lungs are usually ventilated (see Figure 7.3a). At the point that one lung needs to be deflated, the cuff on the bronchial lumen is inflated and ventilation continued into this lung. The proximal end of the shorter lumen is disconnected and ventilation via this lumen is stopped (the tube from

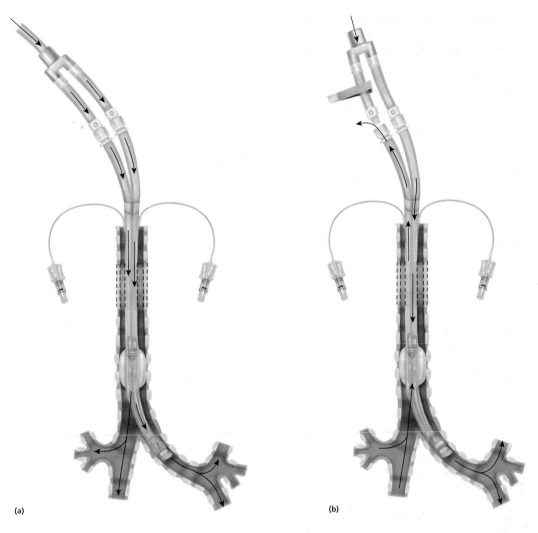

(a)   (b)

Figure 7.3 Left-sided double-lumen tube, arrows showing direction of gas flow. (a) Ventilation of both lungs.
(b) Ventilation of left lung, deflation of right lung.

the ventilator, proximal to the disconnection, must be clamped). The gas in the lung can then escape and the lung collapses (see Figure 7.3b).

A left-sided tube is usually chosen as this is slightly easier to insert into the correct position and less likely to obstruct a lobar bronchus. Right-sided tubes are usually reserved for operations involving the left main bronchus.

One of the main problems of OLV is that it creates a shunt, as blood from the right ventricle is now passing through non-ventilated lung and therefore does not become oxygenated before returning to the systemic circulation, resulting in significant hypoxia. In normal lungs, collapse of the lung reduces the blood flow

through it and reduces the magnitude of the shunt. All that may be required to maintain a normal SpO_2 is an increase in the inspired oxygen concentration. If this fails, or the patient has significant underlying pulmonary disease, there are three options:

- partial reinflation of the collapsed lung and the application of a small amount of continuous positive airway pressure (CPAP) to the lumen with 100% oxygen;
- intermittent reinflation of the lung with 100% oxygen;
- return to two-lung ventilation and use surgical retraction of the lung.

At the end of the surgical procedure, a chest drain is usually inserted to allow drainage of any blood or fluid from the pleural cavity and prevent the formation of a pneumothorax from any gas leak from the lung surface. Finally, the deflated lung must be reinflated. This is usually done by reconnecting the ventilator circuit and ventilating the lungs manually at slightly increased peak inflation pressure to fully re-expand the whole lung.

Anaesthesia for the overweight and obese patient

Prevalence of obesity

Obesity is an increasing problem in modern society, and affects all age groups. In the United Kingdom, 62% of the population is overweight or obese (67% men, 57% women). Because obesity is associated with an increase risk of comorbidities (Table 7.1), it is not surprising that obese people are more likely to need surgery. In the United Kingdom, SOBA (Society for Obesity and Bariatric Anaesthesia) has recently been formed for those with an interest in this group of patients to help disseminate best practice. Much of the content below is based on SOBA guidelines [2.5].

Table 7.1 Comorbidities associated with obesity.

- Hypertension
- Ischaemic heart disease
- Atrial fibrillation
- Type 2 diabetes
- Asthma
- Sleep-disordered breathing:
  - Obstructive sleep apnoea (OSA)
  - Obesity hypoventilation syndrome (OHS)
- Thrombosis:
  - Stroke
  - Venous thromboembolism
- Cancer:
  - Colorectal
  - Prostate
  - Endometrial
  - Breast
- Gastro-oesophageal reflux

A range of surgical procedures is now recognized as effective in helping patients lose weight (bariatric surgery) and anaesthesia for these has become a specialist area; the specifics of this are beyond the scope of this book. The aim here is to outline the principles of managing obese patients safely when they present for anaesthesia and non-bariatric surgery, for example hernia repair, hip replacement.

Preoperative assessment

The specifics of preoperative assessment of obese patients are covered in Chapter 2.

Anaesthesia

As with all non-routine situations, proper planning and preparation are essential.

Equipment and logistics

Consider the following as a minimum:

- appropriate operating table – must be capable of withstanding the weight and supporting the patient's lateral spread when supine (same applies in the CT scanner);
- padding and supports, restraining straps;
- pressure sore prevention – specialized mattresses;
- calf compressors of an appropriate size;
- correct size blood pressure cuff; have a low threshold for intra-arterial blood pressure monitoring;
- ramping pillow (Figure 7.4);

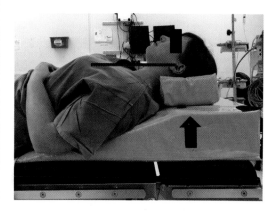

Figure 7.4 Ramping pillow used to facilitate laryngoscopy and intubation. The horizontal line indicates the optimal head extension with the external auditory meatus level with the sternum.

- difficult airway equipment;
- long needles for regional and nerve blocks;
- appropriate mechanical ventilator – capable of pressure modes and positive end expiratory pressure (PEEP);
- adequate numbers of trained staff to move the patient;
- consider:
  - self-positioning by patient prior to induction of anaesthesia;
  - induction of anaesthesia on the operating table in theatre.

Aspects of anaesthesia

- Preoxygenation is less effective due to reduced FRC. Head-up tilt may be preferable to supine.
- To calculate the correct drug dose, four 'weights' are used (Table 7.2), as body composition affects how drugs are distributed between water and fat and hence their effect and elimination:
  - total body weight (TBW);
  - ideal body weight (IBW):
    - males: height (cm) – 100
    - females: height (cm) – 105
  - lean body weight (LBW): calculated from a nomogram using height (cm) and weight (kg). This exceeds ideal body weight in the obese and plateaus at
    $\approx 100\,kg$ for males and $\approx 70\,kg$ for females;
  - adjusted body weight (ABW):
    ABW = IBW + 0.4 (TBW – IBW).
- Venous thromboembolism (VTE) prophylaxis during surgery with preoperative low molecular weight heparin (LMWH) and intraoperative mechanical calf compressors.
- Assessment and management of blood glucose, especially if patient is diabetic and/or during a long operation.
- Airway management: rapid desaturation may occur at induction. These patients will not maintain adequate spontaneous ventilation when anaesthetized and are at increased risk of regurgitation and aspiration, therefore intubation and positive pressure ventilation is preferred. For most patients, standard laryngoscopy and tracheal intubation is practicable. A short-handled laryngoscope can prove very useful if there is limited room between the patient's chin and chest wall when positioned. Aim for the tragus at the level of the sternum using a ramping pillow (see Figure 7.4). Consider awake, fibreoptic intubation in patients who are hypoxaemic at rest or in whom there are additional features suggesting difficult facemask ventilation or direct laryngoscopy. PEEP during ventilation will help to maintain alveolar recruitment and hence oxygenation.
- Minimising postoperative respiratory depression:
  - use short-acting drugs, e.g. desflurane, propofol infusion, remifentanil;
  - maximize use of non-opioid analgesia and regional anaesthetic techniques;
  - at the end of anaesthesia, ensure full reversal of neuromuscular block;
  - extubate awake, with the patient sat as upright as possible;
- give multimodal postoperative nausea and vomiting (PONV) prophylaxis.

Table 7.2 Suggested drug doses.

Lean body weight (males 100 kg, females 70 kg)	Adjusted body weight (ideal plus 40% excess)
Propofol (induction)	Propofol (infusion)
Thiopentone	Alfentanil
Fentanyl	
Morphine	Antibiotics
Bupivacaine/lidocaine	Low molecular weight heparin
Rocuronium	Neostigmine (max. 5 mg)
Atracurium	Sugammadex
Vecuronium	
Paracetamol	
Suxamethonium – use total body weight	

Postoperative care

- Keep patients sat upright.
- Aim for oxygen saturations as preoperative, and monitor SpO_2 continuously. Patients who use CPAP at home, who suffer significant sleep apnoea or arterial desaturation may also benefit from postoperative CPAP immediately after extubation. This may need to be maintained for several days postoperatively.
- Where possible avoid long-acting opioids, but use non-steroidal anti-inflammatory drugs (NSAIDs) with care to avoid the risk of renal failure. VTE prophylaxis may be needed for an extended period. Early mobilization is essential.
- Have a low threshold for providing postoperative care in a high-dependency unit (HDU) in order to achieve all the above.

Anaesthesia for children

Anaesthetizing children can be very challenging as a result of their physiological, anatomical and emotional differences compared with adults [7.5]. In addition, it is now standard practice to allow parents to be involved in their child's treatment at all stages, including during the induction of and recovery from anaesthesia.

Consent

In the United Kingdom, 16 is the age of legal consent although this extends to 18 in special circumstances, except in some parts of the United Kingdom (Scotland). Below the age of 16, consent to medical treatment for children born in England, Wales or Northern Ireland can only be given by adults with parental responsibility for the child (Table 7.3). If the child is close to the age of 16, and deemed to be emotionally and intellectually competent to consent for the proposed treatment themselves, then they are called 'Gillick' or 'Fraser' competent and can be involved in the consent process. If there is any doubt about responsibility, expert advice is essential.

Although it is generally discouraged to think of children as small adults, it is reasonable to recognize that most anaesthetic techniques used in adult anaesthetic practice can be used equally successfully in children but with scaled-down equipment. The main exception to this is the use of regional techniques, with the patient awake, although some spinal anaesthetics are used on very premature babies in specialist centres.

Although the term 'child' is generally used for all ages, the following terms are more widely accepted:

- neonate – birth to 28 days or up to 44 weeks post conception if premature;
- infant – 28 days to 12 months;
- child – 1 year to puberty.

Anatomical and physiological considerations

Children are physically smaller and all of their physiological systems are immature when compared to adults. Of greatest relevance to the anaesthetist are the differences in the respiratory and cardiovascular systems.

Table 7.3 Parental responsibility.

Individual	Degree of responsibility
Mother	Automatic from birth
Father married to the mother	Automatic from birth
Unmarried father	If named on the birth certificate for a child born after a specific date*
	If he has obtained legal responsibility by:
	• joint registration of birth with mother after a specific date*
	• a parental responsibility agreement with mother
	• a parental responsibility order from a court
Same-sex partners	Both, if civil partners at time of treatment
Adoptive parent	Once adoption formalized

*Dependent on which part of the UK born in [7.7].

Anatomical differences

Children have several anatomical features that can make their tracheal intubation more difficult for those who are relatively inexperienced [7.6].

- They have comparatively larger heads. Pillows are rarely needed to obtain the optimal intubation position and the classic 'sniffing the morning air' position used in adult practice.
- They have a large tongue that may compromise the view of the larynx.
- The epiglottis is larger and 'floppy' and tends to obscure a clear view of the larynx. As a result, the laryngoscope blades used are often straighter and placed posterior to the epiglottis in an attempt to elevate it out of the field of vision.
- The narrowest region of a child's airway is at the level of the cricoid ring, compared to the laryngeal inlet in an adult. Consequently, cuffed tracheal tubes are not necessary to obtain a seal. Until recently, cuffed tracheal tubes were considered inappropriate for use in prepubertal children for fear of trauma from the cuff causing swelling and compromise of the airway on extubation. Many experienced paediatric anaesthetists are now using specially designed micro-cuffed tracheal tubes, although great care must be taken in patient selection, tube positioning and cuff inflation.
- A number of different formulas are used to calculate the correct tracheal tube size, both diameter and length. None is proven to be more accurate than any other. In the United Kingdom, the formula from the Advanced Paediatric Life Support (APLS) course is widely used (Table 7.4).

Physiological differences

- A propensity to desaturate much more quickly than adults if oxygenation is interrupted. This is because their lung volume at the end of expiration (FRC) is comparatively very small and contains a smaller 'reservoir' of oxygen.
- They have a higher oxygen consumption per kilogram body weight and consume stored oxygen startlingly quickly.
- The resting heart rate of children of all ages is much higher than that of adults. This requires the anaesthetist to be aware of what is normal at any given age of child. The cardiac output in infants is directly related to their heart rate and they can only increase their cardiac output by increasing their heart rate. A heart rate of less than 60/minute

Table 7.4 Useful paediatric formulas.

Age	
Formulas to estimate weight (kg)	
0–12 months	(Age/2)+4
1–5 years	(Age×2)+8
6–12 years	(Age×3)+7
Formulas to estimate ETT size	
Tracheal tube size internal diameter (mm)	(Age/4)+4
Tracheal tube length (cm) at lips (oral intubation)	(Age/2)+12
Tracheal tube length (cm) at lips (nasal intubation)	(Age/2)+15

ETT, endotracheal tube.

in infants will compromise output to the extent that it is considered life threatening and treated as if they are in asystole, with full cardiorespiratory resuscitation.
- Normal blood pressure values are lower in children and only increase to adult levels by the time they reach their late teens.

As drug doses are given on a per kilogram body weight basis, accurate measurement of body weight is essential prior to anaesthesia. As in adults, lean body weight rather than actual weight should be used in obese children. In situations where it may not be possible to weigh a child, e.g. an emergency, an estimate based on age or height can be used. In the United Kingdom, the APLS formula is widely used (see Table 7.4).

Children are intolerant of prolonged periods of starvation, both emotionally and physiologically. They become distressed when denied food and drink and do not have the ability to maintain blood glucose concentrations because of reduced carbohydrate storage as glycogen. Special consideration should be given to keeping any period of preoperative starvation to a minimum. This can be achieved by operating on children first on a mixed list or by minimizing fasting duration; the 2-4-6 rule is a useful guide.

Period of starvation before induction of anaesthesia:

- 2 hours – water and other clear fluids;
- 4 hours – breast milk;
- 6 hours – formula milk, cow's milk or solids.

Commonly used anaesthetic techniques

Anaesthesia can be induced by either the use of intravenous drugs or by inhalational induction, for example using sevoflurane. Whichever technique is chosen, it is virtually universally accepted that one or both parents accompany the child to the anaesthetic room and wait with them until consciousness is lost. The choice of induction is best established by the anaesthetist after discussion with the parents and child. It rarely needs to be a decision imposed on the child unless there is concern about airway patency, in which case inhalational induction is preferred.

Nitrous oxide is still often used as part of the inhalation gas mixture as its presence will increase the rate of uptake of the volatile drugs and thereby the speed of loss of consciousness. If an intravenous induction is preferred, prior application of a local anaesthetic cream over the chosen vein is mandatory in all but the most urgent cases. Ametop (amethocaine 4%) has the advantages of a rapid onset, causes local vasodilatation and its action persists for several hours. It should not be left in contact with the skin for more than 40–60 minutes as it is irritant. The alternative, EMLA, is non-irritant but may cause local vasoconstriction, is slower to work and its effects wear off quickly after it is removed from the skin.

Intravenous cannulas used in paediatrics are necessarily small, usually either 22 G or 24 G (Neoflon™). Their small calibre results in an increased resistance to flow and very slow infusion rates. As fluids are always carefully given using volumetric pumps, in practice this is not usually a problem.

Anaesthesia is maintained, as in adults, by a balanced technique of general anaesthesia with a regional block if at all possible. Most of the blocks familiar from adult anaesthesia can be employed. One technique not often seen in adult practice but frequently used in children is the caudal block. This is an alternative route to deliver drugs into the epidural space via the sacral hiatus; although it significantly reduces the risk of a dural puncture, its low approach tends to block sacral, lumbar and low thoracic nerve roots. Its main use is for lower limb, perineal, groin and low abdominal surgery, either as a single injection technique or as a continuous infusion via an indwelling catheter. In addition to local anaesthetic drugs, clonidine and ketamine may be given to increase the duration of pain relief.

Complications of anaesthesia in children

Many of the complications that have been described in adults also occur in children. One specific complication that is particularly worrying in children is laryngospasm, and as they have small reserves of oxygen they can become profoundly hypoxic very quickly which if untreated may cause cardiac arrest. It is caused by suppression of the laryngeal reflexes, protecting the airway from aspiration of food and secretions, by the anaesthetic drugs used. During recovery from anaesthesia, unless the laryngeal functions that allow us to speak, swallow and cough have returned, any threat to aspiration will cause closure of the vocal cords and laryngospasm. Laryngospasm results from stimulation of the larynx at an intermediate depth of anaesthesia; the child is neither deep enough to overcome the closing reflex nor sufficiently recovered to ensure the reflexes allow them to breathe properly.

Treatment involves prompt restoration of oxygenation via a tightly fitting facemask with CPAP, and if necessary giving an IV induction drug, e.g. propofol, to deepen anaesthesia. An alternative is to give a dose of suxamethonium to rapidly abolish muscle tone and hence the adduction of the vocal cords. This then allows oxygenation and reintubation. In all cases, careful pharyngeal suction should be used to remove the offending secretions.

In general, all children are recovered in a dedicated recovery area to allow parental contact to be re-established as soon as consciousness returns. Most elective paediatric surgery conducted outside of specialist centres is amenable to same-day discharge provided that the child can be given adequate analgesia at home and they have successfully consumed both liquids and solids before discharge. Even in the dedicated children's hospitals, many children are operated and anaesthetized as day cases, the main exception to this being very young or ex-premature babies who are at increased risk of life-threatening apnoea even after the briefest of general anaesthetics.

FURTHER INFORMATION

Allman K, McIndoe A, Wilson I (eds). *Emergencies in Anaesthesia*, 2nd edn. Oxford: Oxford University Press, 2009.

[7.1] http://onlinelibrary.wiley.com/doi/10.1111/anae.12057/pdf
The principles and conduct of anaesthesia for emergency surgery, 2013.
[7.2] http://nice.org.uk/CG132
NICE guidelines for the management of patients undergoing caesarean section, including anaesthetic recommendations.
[7.3] www.oaa-anaes.ac.uk/
The Obstetric Anaesthetists' Association web site.

[7.4] www.thoracic-anesthesia.com
American site, lots of references and great bronchoscopy simulator.

[7.5] www.apagbi.org.uk/
Association of Paediatric Anaesthetists of Great Britain and Ireland web site. Lots of information about all aspects of paediatric anaesthesia.

[7.6] www.das.uk.com/guidelines/paediatric-difficult-airway-guidelines
Paediatric difficult airway guidelines from the DAS.

[7.7] www.gov.uk/parental-rights-responsibilities/what-is-parental-responsibility
UK government web site with full details of parental rights and responsibilities.

8

Recovery from anaesthesia

Learning objectives

After reading this chapter you should understand the principles of:

- ☐ Management of patients during recovery from anaesthesia
- ☐ Monitoring vital signs during recovery from anaesthesia
- ☐ Recognition of hypoxaemia
- ☐ Recognition of impaired ventilation
- ☐ Assessment of postoperative pain
- ☐ Observation of patients who have had regional anaesthesia and managing their ongoing postoperative analgesia
- ☐ Recognition and treatment of the side-effects of epidural and spinal anaesthesia
- ☐ Postoperative fluid management

Apply this knowledge when practising the following skills:

- ☐ Maintaining the airway of a patient recovering from general anaesthesia
- ☐ Giving oxygen using appropriate devices and flows to prevent hypoxaemia
- ☐ Supporting ventilation if inadequate
- ☐ Assessing patients for signs and causes of hypotension
- ☐ Starting treatment of hypotension based upon its cause
- ☐ Planning postoperative fluid therapy for patients undergoing minor and major surgery
- ☐ Assessing patients' postoperative pain and planning treatment

The vast majority of patients recover from anaesthesia and surgery uneventfully but a small and unpredictable number suffer complications. It is now accepted that all patients should be nursed by trained staff, in an area with appropriate facilities to deal with any of the problems that may arise while recovering from anaesthesia [8.1]. Such specialized areas are referred to as the postanaesthesia care unit (PACU) or recovery unit. Most patients will be nursed on a trolley capable of being tipped head down. Patients who have undergone prolonged surgery or where a prolonged

Clinical Anaesthesia: Lecture Notes, Fifth Edition. Matthew Gwinnutt and Carl Gwinnutt.
© 2017 John Wiley & Sons, Ltd. Published 2017 by John Wiley & Sons, Ltd.
Companion website: www.lecturenoteseries.com/anaesthesia

stay in PACU is expected may be nursed on their beds to minimize the number of transfers. Some patients who have undergone specialist surgery – for example, cardiac surgery patients – may be taken directly to a critical care area. The overall aim should be to ensure that patients are comfortable and stable before transfer to the next stage of their care.

The postanaesthesia care unit

Each patient in the PACU should be cared for in a bay equipped with:

- oxygen supply and appropriate delivery systems;
- suction;
- electrocardiogram (ECG) monitoring;
- pulse oximeter;
- non-invasive blood pressure monitor.

In addition, the following must be available immediately.

- *Airway equipment*: oral and nasal airways, a range of tracheal tubes, laryngoscopes, a bronchoscope and the instruments to perform a cricothyroidotomy and tracheostomy. This is usually all contained within an organized 'airway trolley'.
- *Breathing and ventilation equipment*: self-inflating bag-valve-masks, a mechanical ventilator and a chest drain set.
- *Circulation equipment*: a defibrillator, drugs for cardiopulmonary resuscitation (CPR), a range of intravenous (IV) solutions, pressure infusers and devices for IV access.
- *Drugs*: for resuscitation and anaesthesia. Many areas also store dantrolene for treating malignant hyperthermia (see Chapter 4) and lipid emulsion for treatment of local anaesthetic toxicity (see Chapter 6).
- *Additional monitoring equipment*: pressure transducers and a monitor capable of displaying two or three pressure waveforms, an end-tidal carbon dioxide monitor and a thermometer. These may be needed for patients who have undergone complex surgery with invasive monitoring that is continued in the immediate postoperative period or occasionally for those who require resuscitation.

Discharge of the patient

The anaesthetist's responsibility to the patient does not end with termination of the anaesthetic. Although care is handed over to the PACU staff (nurse or equivalent),

Table 8.1 Minimum criteria for discharge from the postanaesthesia care unit.

- Fully conscious and able to maintain own airway (although patient may still be 'sleepy')
- Adequate breathing
- Stable cardiovascular system, with minimal bleeding from the surgical site
- Adequate pain relief
- Normothermic (>36.5 °C)

the responsibility ultimately remains with the anaesthetist until the patient is discharged from the PACU. If there are inadequate numbers of PACU staff to care for a newly admitted patient, the anaesthetist should adopt this role.

 KEY POINT

- A patient who cannot maintain his/her own airway should never be left alone.

The length of time any patient spends in PACU will depend upon a variety of factors, including duration and type of surgery, anaesthetic technique, and the occurrence of any complications. Most units have a policy determining the minimum length of stay (usually around 30 minutes), and agreed discharge criteria (Table 8.1).

Postoperative complications and their management

Hypoxaemia

This is the most important respiratory complication after anaesthesia and surgery. It may start at recovery and in some patients persists for three days or more after surgery. The presence of cyanosis is very insensitive and, when detectable, means the arterial PO_2 will be <8 kPa (55 mmHg), corresponding to a haemoglobin saturation of 85%. Pulse oximetry has had a major impact on the prevention of hypoxaemia and should be used routinely in all patients. If hypoxaemia is severe or persistent, or when there is any doubt, arterial blood gas analysis should be performed.

Hypoxaemia can be caused by a number of factors, either alone or in combination:

- alveolar hypoventilation;
- ventilation and perfusion mismatch within the lungs;
- diffusion hypoxia;
- pulmonary diffusion defects.

Alveolar hypoventilation

This is a common cause of hypoxaemia after general anaesthesia. It is caused by a degree of respiratory depression leading to an insufficient clearance of the CO_2 generated by metabolism. The concentration of CO_2 in the blood and hence alveoli rises (Figure 8.1). This mixes with the inhaled gas mixture, effectively reducing the fraction of gas that is O_2 in the alveoli. As a result, alveolar PO_2 (PAO_2) and arterial PO_2 (PaO_2) fall. In most patients, increasing their inspired oxygen concentration will restore both.

This is the rationale for giving all patients who have had a general anaesthetic supplemental oxygen therapy. Figure 8.2 shows the variation of PaO_2 with ventilation (minute volume). Note the effect of giving 30% oxygen to a patient whose ventilation is 2 L/minute (normally 5 L/minute); the PaO_2 rises from being barely adequate to supranormal. This is because 30% oxygen contains nearly 1.5 times the concentration of oxygen that is in air and can raise PAO_2 to adequate levels. If ventilation is further reduced, a point is eventually reached where there is only ventilation of the anatomical 'dead space' – that is, the volume of the airways that plays no part in gas exchange. If this occurs, irrespective of the inspired oxygen concentration, no oxygen reaches the alveoli and profound hypoxaemia will follow. Note that hyperventilation can only increase oxygenation minimally. This is because it does not alter the main determinant of alveolar oxygen tension, the inspired PO_2.

Common causes of hypoventilation include the following.

- *Obstruction of the airway*: most often secondary to a reduced level of consciousness but also may be due to vomit, blood, or swelling (for example, post thyroid surgery). Partial obstruction causes noisy breathing; in complete obstruction there is little noise despite vigorous efforts. Both will be accompanied by a characteristic 'see-saw' or paradoxical pattern of ventilation, depending on the degree of obstruction. A tracheal tug may also be seen. The risk of airway obstruction can be reduced by recovering a patient in the lateral position, particularly when recovering from surgery where there is a risk of bleeding into the airway (as in ear, nose and throat (ENT) surgery) or regurgitation (bowel obstruction or a history of reflux). If it is not possible to turn the patient (for instance, after a hip replacement), perform a chin lift or jaw thrust (see Chapter 5). An oropharyngeal or nasopharyngeal airway may be required to help maintain the airway in those who are unconscious (see Chapter 5). This group of patients require close monitoring. As the patient recovers and begins to obey commands, they can be sat up at 30° if it is safe to do so.

 KEY POINT

- No patient should be handed to the care of the PACU staff with noisy respiration of unknown cause.

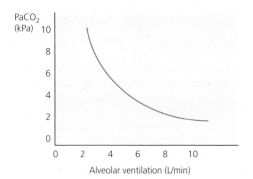

Figure 8.1 Graph showing the relationship between $PaCO_2$ and alveolar ventilation.

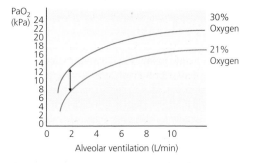

Figure 8.2 Graph showing the relationship between PaO_2 and alveolar ventilation at two different inspired oxygen concentrations.

- *Central respiratory depression*: this is usually due to drugs given during anaesthesia. Both anaesthetic drugs and opioid analgesics depress the normal increase in ventilation seen in response to hypercapnia and hypoxia, and the residual effects of these drugs are commonly present in the recovery period. If ventilation is inadequate, it may need to be supported until the effects of the drugs have worn off or, in the case of severe opioid-induced respiratory depression, the specific antagonist naloxone may be given (see Chapter 4).
- *Impaired mechanics of ventilation*: pain, particularly after upper abdominal or thoracic surgery, prevents coughing, leading to sputum retention and atelectasis. The solution to this is provision of adequate analgesia (consider central neural block). Residual neuromuscular blockade causes weakness and impaired ventilation. The patient will usually show signs of unsustained, jerky movements with rapid, shallow breathing, hypertension and tachycardia. The diagnosis may be confirmed by using a peripheral nerve stimulator, which may show evidence of fade with a train-of-four stimulus (see Chapter 3). The patient should be given oxygen, reassured, sat upright to improve the efficiency of ventilation, and a (further) dose of neostigmine and an anticholinergic given. If rocuronium has been given, sugammadex may be used.
- *Diaphragmatic splinting*: abdominal distension and obesity cause the diaphragm to be pushed into the thorax and increase the work of breathing. Sitting these patients up helps them greatly.
- *Cerebral haemorrhage or ischaemia*: may cause direct damage to the respiratory centre or, more commonly, a deeply unconscious patient unable to maintain a patent airway.
- *Pneumothorax or haemothorax*: both will prevent ventilation of the underlying lung and will require the insertion of a chest drain.
- *Hypothermia*: reduces ventilation but, in the absence of any contributing factors, it does not normally compromise ventilation enough to need specific treatment.

Ventilation and perfusion mismatch within the lungs

Normally, alveolar ventilation (V) and perfusion with blood (Q) are well matched (V/Q = 1) and the haemoglobin in blood leaving the lungs is almost fully saturated with oxygen (97–98%). This is disturbed (ventilation/perfusion (V/Q) mismatch) during anaesthesia and the recovery period, with development of areas where:

- *perfusion exceeds ventilation (V/Q < 1)*: haemoglobin leaving these areas of lung will have a reduced oxygen saturation;
- *ventilation exceeds perfusion (V/Q > 1)*: this can be considered wasted ventilation. Only a small additional volume of oxygen is taken up as the haemoglobin is already almost fully saturated.

In the most extreme situation, there is perfusion of areas of the lung but no ventilation (V/Q = 0). Blood leaving these areas remains 'venous' and is often referred to as 'shunted blood' (that is, it is effectively shunted directly from the venous to arterial system). This is then mixed with fully oxygenated blood leaving ventilated areas of the lungs. The net result is:

- blood perfusing alveoli ventilated with air has an oxygen content of approximately 20 mL/100 mL of blood;
- blood perfusing unventilated alveoli remains venous, with an oxygen content of 15 mL/100 mL of blood;
- the final oxygen content of blood leaving the lungs will be dependent on the relative proportions of shunted blood and non-shunted blood.

 KEY POINT

- For an equivalent blood flow, areas of V/Q < 1 decrease oxygen content more than areas of V/Q > 1 can increase it, even if the inspired oxygen concentration is increased to 100%.

The aetiology of V/Q mismatch is multifactorial but the following are recognized as being of importance.

- Mechanical ventilation reduces cardiac output. This reduces perfusion of non-dependent areas of the lungs, whilst maintaining ventilation. This is worst in the lateral position, when the upper lung is better ventilated and the lower lung better perfused.
- A reduced functional residual capacity (FRC). In supine, anaesthetized patients, particularly those over 50 years of age, the FRC falls below their closing capacity – the lung volume below which some airways close and distal alveoli are no longer ventilated. Eventually, areas of atelectasis develop, mainly in dependent areas of the lung, resulting in increased shunt.

- Pain restricts breathing and coughing, leading to poor ventilation of the lung bases, sputum retention, basal atelectasis and, ultimately, infection. The highest incidence of this is seen in the following circumstances:
  - smokers;
  - obesity;
  - pre-existing lung disease;
  - elderly patients;
  - after upper gastrointestinal or thoracic surgery;
  - three days after surgery.

The effects of small areas of V/Q mismatch can be compensated for by increasing the inspired oxygen concentration. However, because of the disproportionate effect of areas where V/Q <1, once more than 30% of the pulmonary blood flow is passing through such areas, even breathing 100% oxygen will not eliminate hypoxaemia. The oxygen content of the blood leaving alveoli ventilated with 100% oxygen will only have increased by 1 mL/100 mL of blood over what was achieved when being ventilated with air (Table 8.2). This is insufficient to offset the reduction caused by areas of low V/Q. Oxygen therapy is relatively ineffective when the cause of hypoxaemia is V/Q mismatch compared to when hypoventilation exists. Treatment should be aimed at optimizing ventilation of collapsed alveoli. The simplest manoeuvre is to sit the patient upright in bed, which relieves upward pressure on the diaphragm, easing the work of breathing and so improving aeration of the lung bases. The next manoeuvre is to apply continuous positive airways pressure (CPAP) via a closely fitting facemask and a suitable circuit. This recruits alveoli but may be poorly tolerated by patients for periods of more than a few hours.

Diffusion hypoxia

Nitrous oxide absorbed during anaesthesia has to be excreted during recovery. It is very insoluble in blood, and so rapidly diffuses down a concentration gradient into the alveoli, where it reduces the partial pressure of oxygen, making the patient hypoxaemic. This can be treated by giving oxygen via a facemask to increase the inspired oxygen concentration (see later in this chapter).

Pulmonary diffusion defects

Any chronic condition causing thickening of the alveolar membrane, such as fibrosing alveolitis, impairs transfer of oxygen into the blood. In the recovery period, it may also occur secondary to the development of pulmonary oedema following fluid overload or impaired left ventricular function. It should be treated by first administering oxygen to increase the partial pressure of oxygen in the alveoli and then by management of any underlying cause.

Management of hypoxaemia

All patients should be given oxygen in the immediate postoperative period to:

- counter the effects of diffusion hypoxia when nitrous oxide has been used;
- compensate for any hypoventilation;
- compensate for V/Q mismatch as much as possible;
- meet the increased oxygen demand when shivering.

The need for and effectiveness of oxygen therapy are best determined either by arterial blood gas analysis or by using a pulse oximeter. Oxygen therapy should follow the British Thoracic Society guidelines [8.2]. Patients who continue to hypoventilate, have persistent

 KEY POINT

- Oxygen therapy is relatively ineffective at relieving hypoxaemia where the cause is V/Q mismatch compared to hypoventilation. Opening (recruiting) unventilated alveoli is likely to be more effective.

Table 8.2 Effect of alveolar oxygen concentration on oxygen content of blood.

	Alveolar oxygen concentration (%)	Haemoglobin saturation (%)	Oxygen content (mL/100 mL blood)
Alveoli containing air	21	97	20
Alveoli containing oxygen	100	100	21
Non-ventilated alveoli	Very low	75	15

V/Q mismatch, are obese, anaemic or have ischaemic heart disease may require additional oxygen for an extended period of time.

KEY POINT

* Aim to maintain the SpO$_2$ between 94% and 98%, unless the patient is known to have severe chronic obstructive pulmonary disease (COPD) when a value of 88–92% is acceptable.

Devices used for delivery of oxygen

Variable-performance devices: masks or nasal cannulas

These are adequate for the majority of patients recovering from anaesthesia and surgery. The precise concentration of oxygen inspired by the patient is unknown as it is dependent upon the patient's respiratory pattern and the flow of oxygen used (usually 2–12 L/minute). The inspired gas consists of a mixture of:

* oxygen flowing into the mask;
* oxygen that has accumulated under the mask during the expiratory pause;
* alveolar gas from the previous breath which has collected under the mask;
* air entrained during peak inspiratory flow from the holes in the side of the mask and from leaks between the mask and face.

The most commonly used device is the Hudson mask (Figure 8.3a). As a guide, it will increase the inspired oxygen concentration to 25–60% with oxygen flows of 2–12 L/minute.

Patients unable to tolerate a facemask who can nose breathe may find either a single foam-tipped catheter or double catheters, placed just inside the vestibule of the nose, more comfortable (Figure 8.3b). Lower flows, 2–4 L/minute, of oxygen are used, which increases the inspired oxygen concentration to 25–40%.

If higher inspired oxygen concentrations are needed in a spontaneously breathing patient, a Hudson mask with a reservoir bag can be used (Figure 8.4a). A one-way valve diverts the oxygen flow into the reservoir during expiration. The contents of the reservoir, along with the high flow of oxygen (12–15 L/minute), can almost meet the demand of peak inspiration gas flow, resulting in minimal entrainment of air, raising the inspired concentration to approximately 85%. An inspired oxygen concentration of 100% can only be achieved by using

either an anaesthetic system with a close-fitting face-mask or a self-inflating bag with reservoir and non-rebreathing valve and an oxygen flow of 12–15 L/minute.

Fixed-performance devices

These are used when it is important to deliver a precise concentration of oxygen, unaffected by the patient's pattern of ventilation, for example patients with COPD and carbon dioxide retention. These masks work on the principle of high-airflow oxygen enrichment (HAFOE). Oxygen is fed into a Venturi

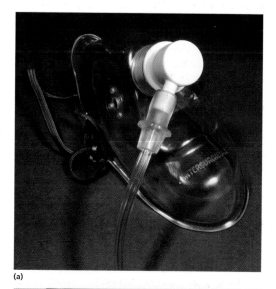
(a)

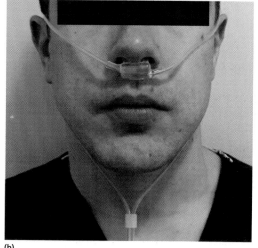
(b)

Figure 8.3 (a) Hudson mask. (b) Nasal catheters in position.

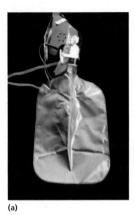 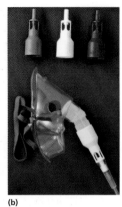

(a)　　　　　　　　　　　(b)

Figure 8.4 (a) Hudson mask with reservoir. (b) High-airflow oxygen enrichment (HAFOE; Venturi) mask.

that entrains a much greater but constant flow of air. The total flow into the mask should be as high as 45 L/minute. The high gas flow has two effects: it meets the patient's peak inspiratory flow, stopping air being drawn in around the mask, and flushes expiratory gas, reducing rebreathing. Various interchangeable Venturis, each a different colour and delivering a set oxygen concentration (usually 24%, 28%, 35%, 40% and 60%), are available (Figure 8.4b).

The above systems all deliver dry gas to the patient that may cause crusting or thickening of secretions and difficulty with clearance. For prolonged use, a HAFOE system should be used with a humidifier.

High-flow nasal oxygen

This system delivers oxygen at flow rates that exceed patients' peak inspiratory flow rate (>50 L/minute), thereby delivering a known concentration of oxygen, similar to the Venturi facemask but via nasal cannulas. Unlike when the simple nasal cannulas (see Figure 8.3b) are used, these high flow rates are well tolerated as the oxygen is warmed to 37 °C and humidified (to 100% relative humidity) before entering the respiratory tract.

Hypotension

This can be due to a variety of factors, alone or in combination:

- a reduction in circulating volume (preload);
- a reduced cardiac output (reduced myocardial contractility, valvular dysfunction, arrhythmias);
- vasodilatation (afterload).

These should be assessed and treated using a step-wise approach.

Step 1: Assess the circulating volume (preload)

Hypovolaemia is the commonest cause of hypotension after anaesthesia and surgery. Although intraoperative blood loss is usually obvious, continued bleeding, especially in the absence of surgical drains, may not be. Fluid loss may also occur as a result of tissue damage leading to oedema, or from evaporation during prolonged surgery on body cavities, for example the abdomen or thorax (see later). The diagnosis can be confirmed by the following findings.

- Cold clammy skin, delayed capillary refill (>2 seconds) in the absence of fear, pain and hypothermia.
- Tachycardia, with a pulse of poor volume.
- Narrowed pulse pressure; initially, systolic blood pressure may be reduced minimally but the diastolic elevated as a result of compensatory vasoconstriction. The blood pressure must always be interpreted in conjunction with the other assessments.
- Inadequate urine output (<0.3 mL/kg/hour), best measured hourly via a catheter and urometer. Also consider the following as causes of reduced urine output:
  - a blocked catheter (blood clot or lubricant);
  - hypoxia;
  - renal damage intraoperatively (e.g. during aortic aneurysm surgery).

The extent to which these changes occur will depend primarily upon the degree of hypovolaemia. A tachycardia may not be seen in the patient taking beta-blockers, and a fit, young patient may lose up to 15% of their blood volume without detectable signs.

 KEY POINT

- The commonest cause of oliguria is hypovolaemia; anuria is usually due to a blocked catheter.

Treatment

This is covered in detail in Chapter 9.

Step 2: Assess cardiac output

The commonest causes of a reduction in cardiac output with normovolaemia are left ventricular dysfunction due to ischaemic heart disease (or more rarely valvular heart disease) or an arrhythmia.

Left ventricular dysfunction

It is not uncommon to mistake this condition for hypo-volaemia based on the presence of poor peripheral circulation, tachycardia and tachypnoea. However, further examination may reveal:

- distended neck veins, raised jugular venous pressure (JVP);
- basal crepitations on auscultation of the lungs;
- wheeze with a productive cough;
- a triple rhythm on auscultation of the heart.

A chest X-ray may be diagnostic. Echocardiography will demonstrate reduced contractility (hypokinesis) despite adequate ventricular filling suggesting myo-cardial ischaemia.

Treatment

- Sit the patient upright.
- Give 100% oxygen.
- Monitor the ECG, blood pressure and peripheral oxygen saturation.

Further details are given in Chapter 9.

Arrhythmias

Disturbances of cardiac rhythm are a common cause of hypotension and occur more frequently in the presence of:

- hypoxaemia;
- hypovolaemia;
- hypercapnia;
- hypothermia;
- sepsis;
- pre-existing ischaemic heart disease;
- electrolyte abnormalities;
- acid–base disturbances;
- inotropes, antiarrhythmics, bronchodilators.

Correction of the underlying problem will result in spontaneous resolution of many arrhythmias. Specific intervention is required if there is a significant reduc-tion in cardiac output and hypotension. The manage-ment outlined below is based upon the Resuscitation Council (UK) 2015 guidelines.

Tachycardia

Cardiac filling occurs during diastole, which is pro-gressively shortened as the heart rate increases. The result is insufficient time for ventricular filling, lead-ing to a reduced cardiac output and eventually a fall in blood pressure. If the contribution from atrial con-traction is also lost (for example, in atrial fibrillation) there is further compromise. As coronary artery flow is dependent on diastolic time (and diastolic blood pressure), myocardial ischaemia is more likely, par-ticularly in combination with hypotension.

- *Sinus tachycardia (>100 beats/minute)*: this is the commonest arrhythmia after anaesthesia and surgery, usually a result of:
  o pain;
  o hypovolaemia;
  o if there is associated pyrexia, it may be an early indication of sepsis;
  o drugs – anticholinergics, e.g. cyclizine, glycopyrrolate;
  o rarely, it may be the first sign of malignant hyperpyrexia.

Treatment consists of oxygen, analgesia and adequate fluid replacement. If the tachycardia persists, a small dose of a beta-blocker may be given intravenously whilst monitoring the ECG, providing there are no contraindications. Treatment of a supraventricular tachycardia (most commonly atrial fibrillation) is covered in Chapter 9.

Bradycardia

Although a slow heart rate reduces myocardial oxygen demand and allows adequate time for ventricular filling, eventually the point is reached where end-diastolic volume is maximal, and further reductions in heart rate reduce cardiac output and hypotension ensues (remem-ber cardiac output = heart rate × stroke volume).

- *Sinus bradycardia (<60 beats/minute)*: usually the result of:
  o an inadequate dose of an anticholinergic (for instance, glycopyrrolate) given with neostigmine to reverse neuromuscular block;
  o excessive suction to clear pharyngeal or tracheal secretions;
  o excessive high spread of spinal or epidural anaesthesia;
  o the development of an inferior myocardial infarction;
  o excessive beta-blockade preoperatively or intraoperatively.

Treatment should consist of removing any provoking stimuli and giving oxygen. Further details of treat-ment are given in Chapter 9.

Step 3: Assess for vasodilatation

This is common during spinal or epidural anaes-thesia (see Chapter 6), a typical example being after prostate surgery under spinal anaesthesia. As the legs are taken down from the lithotomy position, vasodilatation in the lower limbs is unmasked, and as the patient is moved to the PACU they become profoundly hypotensive. Hypotension secondary to regional anaesthesia is corrected by giving fluids (crystalloid or colloid), vasopressors (for example, ephedrine) or a combination of both. The combination of hypovolaemia and vasodilatation will cause profound hypotension. Oxygen should always be given.

Sometimes the cause of hypotension is multifactorial, as in septic shock. A patient may initially present with peripheral vasodilatation causing hypotension and tachycardia in the absence of blood loss. The patient may be pyrexial and if the cardiac output is measured, it is usually elevated. As sepsis worsens, it can lead to reduced cardiac contractility, worsening hypotension and poor perfusion, leading to an acidosis and arrhythmia, often atrial fibrillation. The diagnosis should be suspected in any patient who has had surgery associated with a septic focus, for example free infection in the peritoneal cavity or where there is infection in the genitourinary tract. This usually presents several hours after the patient has left the PACU, often during the night following daytime surgery. The causative micro-organism is often a Gram-negative bacterium. Patients developing septic shock require early diagnosis, invasive monitoring and circulatory support in a critical care area (see Chapter 9). Antibiotic therapy should be targeted at the suspected causative organism or according to any positive culture results with advice from a microbiologist.

> **KEY POINT**
>
> - When treating hypotension, correct hypovolaemia before using inotropes.

Hypertension

This is commonest in patients with pre-existing hypertension, but may be caused or exacerbated by:

- pain;
- hypoxaemia;
- hypercapnia;
- confusion or delirium;
- hypothermia.

Hypertension with coexisting tachycardia and in the presence of ischaemic heart disease is particularly dangerous as both increase myocardial work and oxygen consumption and may cause an acute myocardial infarction. If the blood pressure remains elevated after correcting the above, a vasodilator or beta-blocker may be necessary. Senior help should be sought.

Postoperative nausea and vomiting (PONV)

This occurs in up to 80% of patients following anaesthesia and surgery. It is rarely fatal, but it is unpleasant and leaves patients feeling dissatisfied with the care they have received. Some patients would rather have pain than PONV. It may cause delayed discharge from hospital and thereby increase costs. For these reasons, it is to be taken seriously and measures should be employed to avoid it.

Patients identified as being at high risk of PONV (Apfel score ≥2 points; see Chapter 2) should be given a combination of two antiemetics before emergence from anaesthesia because it is often easier to prevent vomiting than to stop it once it has started. Failure of treatment may be addressed in the PACU by giving an additional drug from the different classes (see Chapter 4). Most PACUs have a PONV pathway to ensure optimal management of patients at risk (Figure 8.5).

Postoperative intravenous fluid therapy

In 2013, NICE issued clinical guideline 174, Intravenous fluid therapy in adults in hospital [4.4]. This contains recommendations on general principles for IV fluid therapy for a number of situations including routine maintenance, replacement and resuscitation. The guidelines stress the importance of assessment and monitoring that includes history, clinical examination, current medications, fluid balance, weight and appropriate laboratory investigations.

Routine maintenance

This consists of:

- 25–30 mL/kg/day of water;
- 1–1.5 mmol/kg/day of sodium, potassium and chloride;
- 50–100 g/day glucose to limit starvation ketosis;
- for obese patients, calculate requirement based on ideal body weight. Patients rarely need more than 3 L/day;

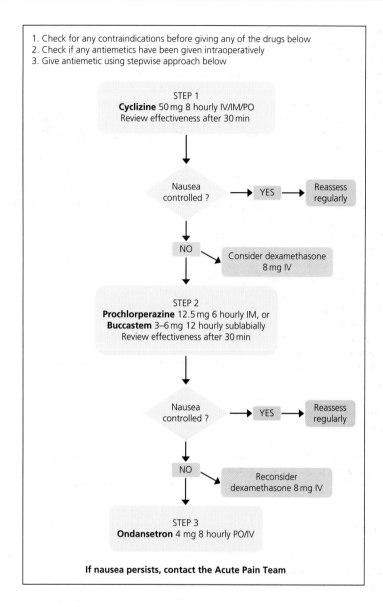

1. Check for any contraindications before giving any of the drugs below
2. Check if any antiemetics have been given intraoperatively
3. Give antiemetic using stepwise approach below

STEP 1
Cyclizine 50 mg 8 hourly IV/IM/PO
Review effectiveness after 30 min

Nausea controlled ? → YES → Reassess regularly

NO → Consider dexamethasone 8 mg IV

STEP 2
Prochlorperazine 12.5 mg 6 hourly IM, or
Buccastem 3–6 mg 12 hourly sublabially
Review effectiveness after 30 min

Nausea controlled ? → YES → Reassess regularly

NO → Reconsider dexamethasone 8 mg IV

STEP 3
Ondansetron 4 mg 8 hourly PO/IV

If nausea persists, contact the Acute Pain Team

Figure 8.5 Treatment pathway for postoperative nausea and vomiting (PONV).

- consider less fluid for patients who:
  - are older or frail;
  - have renal impairment or cardiac failure;
  - are malnourished.

Replacement

Adjust the volume and type of fluid to take into account additional fluid and electrolyte losses or abnormal distribution. Typical losses include:

- vomiting or nasogastric drainage:
  - 20–80 mmol/L Na^+;
  - 14 mmol/L K^+;
  - 140 mmol/L Cl^-;
  - 60–80 mmol/L H^+

(if excessive, can cause a hypochloraemic, hypokalaemic, metabolic alkalosis);

- diarrhoea or colostomy losses:
  - 30–140 mmol/L Na^+;
  - 30–70 mmol/L K^+;
  - 20–80 mmol/L HCO_3^-;

- pancreatic drain or fistula losses:
  - 125–138 mmol/L Na$^+$;
  - 8 mmol/L K$^+$;
  - 56 mmol/L Cl$^-$;
  - 85 mmol/L HCO$_3^-$.

Resuscitation

Use crystalloids that contain sodium in a concentration of 130–154 mmol/L. Give a bolus of 500 mL in less than 15 minutes. There is some evidence that balanced crystalloid solutions (e.g. Hartmann's) may cause less physiological disturbance compared to the use of 0.9% sodium chloride. Gelatins can also be used, and there is some evidence that less volume of fluid may be required when these are used compared to crystalloids. However, colloids alone cannot be used, as some free water must be provided. Human albumin can be considered for use when resuscitating patients with severe sepsis.

Saline is also available as a hypertonic solution consisting of between 1.8% and 7.5% sodium chloride solutions. When given, these raise the osmolality of the extracellular fluid (ECF) (mainly the intravascular component) and create a gradient such that water moves from the intracellular fluid (ICF) into the plasma. The intravascular volume is expanded by a greater volume than the volume of hypertonic solution given, for example 250 mL 7.5% saline results in plasma expansion by up to 1.5 L. If given repeatedly, they will result in intracellular dehydration, which must be corrected subsequently. There is no evidence for their routine use during in the perioperative period but they may have a role in resuscitating patients with traumatic brain injury, where they appear to reduce cerebral oedema, restore cerebral perfusion and help reduce neuronal injury.

Planning postoperative fluid management

Using a 70 kg man as an example, he is composed of approximately 45 L of water, of which 30 L are in the intracellular space and 15 L in the extracellular space. The latter is divided into the interstitial space (10 L) and the intravascular space (5 L). Daily water intake is approximately 2250 mL comprising 1750 mL orally and 500 mL in food. A further 250 mL is generated by the oxidation of carbohydrates. A similar volume is lost each day: 1500 mL as urine, 100 mL in faeces and 900 mL as insensible losses (300 mL via the lungs, 600 mL via the skin). To maintain electrolyte balance, the following intake is required: sodium 70–100 mmol, potassium 70 mmol and 10–15 mmol each of calcium, magnesium and phosphate. Inadequate water intake is sensed by osmo- and volume receptors that stimulate the release of antidiuretic hormone (ADH) and the sensation of thirst.

Minor surgery

All patients having an anaesthetic (and surgery) undergo a period of fasting pre- and intraoperatively, resulting in a water deficit. The loss comes from the total body water (intra- and extracellular fluid), which therefore has little effect on the intravascular volume. Although this is tolerated when surgery is relatively minor and there is no significant blood loss, there is increasing evidence that giving patients IV fluids even during relatively minor surgical procedures (e.g. knee arthroscopy) reduces the incidence of PONV. This is particularly true in children, the elderly and those patients with a high risk of PONV, who are very intolerant of even relatively minor degrees of dehydration where giving fluids reduces the risk of PONV.

If no IV fluid is given and surgery is prolonged, or a patient has failed to drink within 4–6 hours of recovering from anaesthesia, usually as a result of nausea and vomiting, IV fluid will be required. Providing that the volume of vomit is not excessive, only maintenance fluids are required, calculated at 25–30 mL/kg/day, but must take into account the accrued deficit.

For example, the 70 kg patient above, fasted from 08:00 to 14:00, who has had no IV fluid and is still unable to take fluids by mouth at 18:00, will require:

- 25 mL/kg/day to make up the deficit from 08:00 to 18:00:

$$25 \times 70 \times (10/24) = 730 \text{ mL}$$

- 25 mL/kg/day from 18:00 to 08:00 the following morning:

$$25 \times 70 \times (14/24) = 1020 \text{ mL}$$

The total IV fluid requirement = 1750 mL in the next 14 hours if the patient is not able to resume oral intake. An appropriate rate for the IV fluid would be:

- 1000 mL over the first 6 hours;
- 750 mL over the following 7.5 hours.

This should contain the daily requirement of Na$^+$ 1–1.5 mmol/kg and could be given as:

- 1000 mL 5% glucose plus 750 mL Hartmann's.

In practice, most patients would probably be prescribed fluid at the rate of 1000 mL per 8 hours as either 0.9% saline or Hartmann's solution. Clearly, this contains a greater amount of sodium than required, but this is excreted easily by the kidneys. Whatever regime is prescribed, patients should be reviewed at 22:00 and 08:00 the following morning to ensure that they are adequately hydrated (see later in this chapter).

Major surgery

Postoperative fluid balance following major surgery is more complex. Assuming that appropriate volumes of water, electrolytes and blood have been given during the operation, the postoperative fluid and electrolyte requirements will depend upon:

- the volume needed for maintenance, which will be increased if the patient is pyrexial;
- replacement of continuing losses from the gastrointestinal tract, for example via a nasogastric tube, fistulas, diarrhoea;
- losses into drains;
- any continued bleeding;
- rewarming of cold peripheries causing vasodilatation;
- the presence of an epidural for analgesia;
- the extent of tissue trauma or 'third space losses'.

Third space losses

The first and second spaces are the constituents of the ECF, namely the interstitial fluid space and the plasma. These are normal physiological compartments and fluid shifts occur readily between them. A 'third space' related to and formed from the ECF also exists and in non-pathological circumstances is usually referred to as the transcellular water, examples being cerebrospinal fluid (CSF), urine, fluid within the gut, and fluids in the ducts of glands and serous cavities. Accumulation of third space fluid may also be pathological, examples being the swelling of tissues (e.g. after surgical trauma, sepsis or burns) or in 'cavities' (e.g. ascites, pleural effusions and fluid within the bowel lumen in a patient who has an ileus). In health, fluid intake replenishes the ECF but in pathological conditions, the interstitial and plasma fluid volumes become depleted in proportion to the volume of the third space losses. This has a proportionately greater effect on the plasma volume than if the losses were distributed from the total body water, for example in dehydration. The biggest problem for the clinician is that it is impossible to quantify such losses accurately; suffice it to say that the greater the degree of tissue damage from surgery or trauma, the greater the third space losses.

The patient who has undergone major surgery will require close monitoring to ensure that sufficient volumes of the correct fluid are given to replace what has been lost. These losses can be divided into two main groups: those that equate to ECF (blood, losses from the gastrointestinal (GI) tract, third space losses) and those that are mainly water (insensible losses). As seen previously, the former will have a greater immediate effect as a significant part of the loss is from the plasma volume, and consequently will affect the perfusion and oxygenation of vital organs. This must be rectified rapidly. As already mentioned, water losses, unless excessive, have less of an effect on circulating volume and can be replaced more gradually.

In the first 24 hours postoperatively, no single regime can be provided. The adequacy of fluid management is based on good clinical assessment and reassessment, along with appropriate monitoring. The principles described above should be taken into account when calculating and prescribing fluid therapy for each individual patient.

- Maintenance fluids:
  - 25–30 mL/kg/day water, increased by 10% for each °C if the patient is pyrexial;
  - Na^+, 1–1.5 mmol/kg/day;
  - K^+ 1.0 mmol/kg/day.
- Replacement of measured gastrointestinal losses with an equal volume of Hartmann's solution.
- Replacement of ongoing blood loss. Aim for a haemoglobin concentration of 90 g/dL.
  - <500 mL with either Hartmann's solution or 0.9% saline (up to three times the volume of blood lost as crystalloids are distributed throughout the ECF), or colloid, to the same volume as the blood loss;
  - >1000 mL may require transfusion with stored blood.
- Replacement of ongoing losses into the third space.
- Fluid required as a result of epidural-induced vasodilatation.

Patients who have undergone major body cavity surgery may require large volumes of fluid postoperatively. In order to ensure that their demands are met, they must be regularly assessed, clinically, biochemically and by the use of invasive monitoring, where appropriate.

Clinical assessment

- Thirst, dry mucous membranes: early reliable signs of dehydration.
- Cool peripheries, reduced skin turgor, tachycardia, oliguria, drowsiness: imply a significant fluid deficit.
- Hypotension, increased respiratory rate, coma: life threatening.
- Urine output less than 0.5 mL/kg/hour suggests significant hypovolaemia.

Biochemistry

- Raised haematocrit, urea, creatinine: support the diagnosis of dehydration.
- Metabolic acidosis (raised lactate): suggests hypovolaemia and hypoperfusion.

Monitoring

Arterial lines can be inserted easily, and allow the beat-to-beat variation of systolic pressure to be assessed (providing the patient is in sinus rhythm); the greater the variation, the greater the degree of hypovolaemia. This can simply be 'eye-balled' or formally measured using pulse contour analysis, which can also be used to assess cardiac output (see Chapter 3). A low or negative central venous pressure (CVP) has traditionally been interpreted as an indication of fluid depletion but requires the insertion of a central venous catheter. Whichever method is used, trends rather than isolated values are more useful, particularly the response of blood pressure, stroke volume variation and cardiac output to a fluid challenge. Typically, a 250 mL bolus of fluid is given rapidly and the effect noted.

On the second and subsequent days, the same basic principles are used. In addition:

- the fluid balance of the previous 24 hours must be checked;
- ensure that all sources of fluid loss are recorded;
- the patient's serum electrolytes must be checked to ensure adequate replacement and the fluid regime should be adjusted accordingly;
- the urine output for the previous 6 and 24 hours should be noted; if decreasing, consider other causes of fluid loss, such as increasing pyrexia or development of an ileus;
- magnesium and phosphate levels must be checked and replacements given if plasma concentration are low;
- consider starting enteral nutrition, either orally or via a nasogastric tube.

> ### KEY POINT
>
> - A review of the patient's observation charts looking at trends is often more useful than a 'snapshot' of their condition. Deterioration suggests that treatment is inadequate or that there are new or ongoing unidentified problems.

The stress response

Following major surgery and trauma, matters are complicated further. Various neuroendocrine responses result in increased secretion of a variety of hormones, which have an effect on fluid balance. ADH secretion is maximal during surgery and may remain elevated for several days. The effect of this is to increase water absorption by the kidneys and reduce urine output. Aldosterone secretion is raised and, together with activation of the renin–angiotensin system, results in sodium and fluid retention and increased urinary excretion of potassium. Consequently, in some patients, urine output may be as low as 0.5 mL/kg/hour during the first two postoperative days without signifying organ hypoperfusion. Furthermore, they will not have the clinical signs associated with dehydration (see Chapter 9). Additional fluid, in an attempt to restore urine output, is unnecessary and simply leads to greater sodium and water retention, worsening tissue oedema without producing an increase in urine output. This is particularly true after pulmonary and oesophageal surgery, where it has been shown that maintaining normal fluid input and accepting a lower urine output results in fewer postoperative complications, as a result of less tissue oedema and fewer anastomotic breakdowns. It is important to remember that all clinical parameters need to be considered when trying to judge intravascular volume and tissue perfusion. However, in some cases where there are ongoing third space losses, for example after major trauma, patients will exhibit clinical symptoms and signs of fluid depletion and increased IV fluids will be required to maintain an adequate intravascular volume.

After 3–5 days, hormone levels return to normal and this is followed by an increase in the volume of urine passed, which may be augmented as fluid sequestered to the pathological third space is reclaimed.

Postoperative analgesia

After injury, acute pain limits activity until healing has taken place. Modern surgical treatment restores function more rapidly, a process facilitated by the elimination of postoperative pain [8.3]. A good example is the internal fixation of fractures, followed by potent analgesia allowing early mobilization. Ineffective treatment of postoperative pain not only delays this process, but also has other important consequences:

- physical immobility:
  - reduced cough leading to sputum retention and pneumonia;
  - muscle wasting, skin breakdown and cardiovascular deconditioning;
  - thromboembolic disease – deep venous thrombosis and pulmonary embolus;
  - delayed bone and soft tissue healing;
- psychological reaction:
  - reluctance to undergo further, necessary surgical procedures;
- economic costs:
  - prolonged hospital stay, increased medical complications;
  - increased time away from normal occupations;
- development of chronic pain syndromes.

Sometimes pain is a useful aid to diagnosis and must be recognized and acted upon, for example:

- due to a compartment syndrome, or dressings becoming too tight;
- infection from cellulitis, peritonitis or pneumonia;
- referred visceral pain in myocardial infarction (arm or neck) or pancreatitis (to the back).

 KEY POINT

- Any patient who complains of pain that unexpectedly increases in severity, changes in nature or site, or is of new onset should be examined to identify the cause rather than simply being prescribed analgesia.

Factors affecting the experience of pain

Pain and the patient's response to it are very variable and should be understood against the background of the individual's previous personal experiences and expectations rather than compared with the norm.

- Anxiety heightens the experience of pain. The preoperative visit by the anaesthetist plays a significant role in allaying anxiety by explaining what to expect postoperatively, what types of analgesia are available and also by exploring patients' concerns with them.
- Patients who have a pre-existing chronic pain problem are vulnerable to suffering with additional acute pain. Their nervous systems can be considered to be sensitized to pain and will react more strongly to noxious stimuli. Previously bad pain experiences in hospital or anticipation of severe pain for another reason suggest that extra effort will be required to control the pain.
- Older patients tend to require lower doses of analgesics as a result of changes in drug distribution, metabolism, excretion and co-existing disease. Prescribing should take these factors into account rather than using them as an excuse for inadequate analgesia. There is no difference between the intensity of pain suffered by the different sexes having the same operation.
- All patients undergoing surgery should have adequate pain control to allow early mobilization. Upper abdominal and thoracic surgery may cause severe pain in the early postoperative period and good analgesia is likely to have a significant positive impact by improving respiratory function and reducing the risks of sputum retention and infection. Patients undergoing other types of surgery, e.g. knee replacement, may have significant pain for a much longer duration postoperatively with an impact on mobilization. Pain following surgery on the body surface or periphery of limbs is generally less severe and lasts for a shorter duration.

Management of postoperative pain

This can be divided into a number of steps:

- assessment of pain;
- analgesic drugs used;
- techniques of administration;
- difficult pain problems.

Assessment of acute pain

Regular measurement of pain means that it is less likely to be ignored and the efficacy of interventions can be assessed. There are a variety of methods of assessing pain; Table 8.3 shows a simple, practical

Table 8.3 A simple practical scoring system for acute pain.

Pain score	Staff view	Patient's view	Action
0	None	Insignificant or no pain	Consider reducing dose or changing to weaker analgesic, e.g. morphine to NSAID plus paracetamol
1	Mild	In pain, but expected and tolerable; no reason to seek (additional) treatment	Continue current therapy, review regularly
2	Moderate	Unpleasant situation; treatment desirable but not necessarily at the expense of severe treatment side-effects	Continue current therapy, consider additional regular simple analgesia, e.g. paracetamol and/or NSAID
3	Severe	Intolerable situation – will consider even unpleasant treatments to reduce pain	Increase dose of opioid or start opioid; consider alternative technique, e.g. epidural

NSAID, non-steroidal anti-inflammatory drug.

system that is understood by patients and easily applied by staff. The numeric score is to facilitate recording and allows trends to be identified. Pain must be assessed with appropriate activity for the stage of recovery; for example, five days after a hip joint replacement, a patient would not be expected to have pain while lying in bed, but adequate analgesia should allow mobilization with only mild to insignificant pain.

Multimodal analgesia

This is the use of multiple interventions, usually drug based, each of which targets a different step in pain transmission (Figure 8.6). In this way, the synergistic actions provide more effective pain relief with fewer side-effects than a single drug or technique. The combination used will have to take into account:

- the surgical procedure, e.g. gastrointestinal, orthopaedic;
- the patient – co-morbidities, current medications, allergies;
- side-effects of drugs and techniques used, e.g. limb weakness with epidural analgesia;
- point in recovery after surgery.

Commonly used drugs and techniques include:

- opioids;
- non-steroidal anti-inflammatory drugs (NSAIDs);
- paracetamol;
- gabapentinoids;
- N-methyl-D-aspartate (NMDA) receptor antagonists, most commonly ketamine;
- regional/local anaesthetics.

The pharmacology of these drugs and their side-effects are covered in Chapter 4. Their sites of action are shown in Figure 8.6.

Examples of multimodal techniques for surgery and enhanced recovery

- Total knee replacement:
  - preoperative – gabapentin or COX-2 inhibitor;
  - intraoperative – IV paracetamol +/– NSAID +/– dexamethasone. General anaesthesia with IV opioids, or spinal with local anaesthetic (LA) only. High-volume LA wound infiltration;
  - early postoperative – oral opioids (immediate and modified release); IV paracetamol, oral NSAID;
  - late postoperative – oral paracetamol, weak opioid, oral NSAID.
- Laparotomy:
  - preoperative – gabapentin;
  - intraoperative – IV opioids +/– transversus abdominis plane (TAP) or rectus sheath block or; epidural LA plus opioid, IV paracetamol; dexamethasone;
  - early postoperative – low-dose epidural LA or; wound infusion with LA via a catheter, IV paracetamol;
  - late postoperative – oral opioids, oral paracetamol.
- Day-case surgery, e.g. hernia repair:
  - preoperative – oral NSAID;
  - intraoperative – low-dose opioid, IV paracetamol, wound infiltration;
  - postoperative – oral NSAID, regular oral paracetamol.

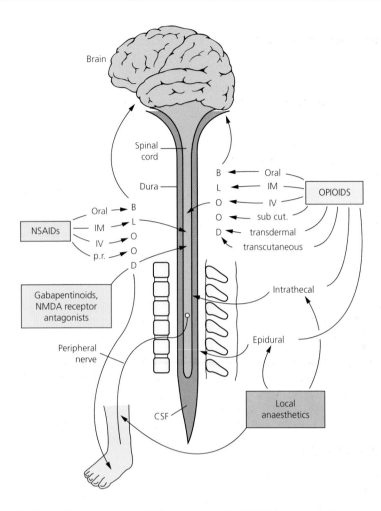

Figure 8.6 Sites of actions of analgesic drugs. CSF, cerebrospinal fluid; IM, intramuscular; IV, intravenous; NMDA, N-methyl-D-aspartate; NSAID, non-steroidal anti-inflammatory.

As can be seen from the above, opioids remain key in the management of postoperative pain. The dose required to achieve this may vary enormously between patients as a result of differences in the following.

- Pharmacodynamics: the effect of the drug on the body (via the receptors).
- Pharmacokinetics: how the body distributes, metabolizes and eliminates the drug.
- The nature of the stimulus.
- The psychological reaction to the situation.

The biggest step forward in the treatment of acute pain with opioids has been the recognition that individual requirements are very variable and the dose needs to be titrated for each patient:

- there is no minimum or maximum dose;
- even with best practice some pain will remain;
- minimum levels of monitoring and intervention are necessary for safe and effective use;
- use a multimodal approach to minimize the dose of opioids and thereby side-effects;
- additional methods of analgesia should be considered if opioid requirements are high.

Analgesic techniques used postoperatively

Patient-controlled analgesia (PCA)

- A microprocessor-controlled syringe pump capable of being programmed is used to deliver a predetermined dose of a drug intravenously.

- Activation is by the patient depressing a switch that is designed to prevent accidental triggering (hence 'patient-controlled').
- To prevent an overdose being given:
  - the maximum dose in any period and any background infusion is predetermined;
  - after successful administration of a dose, a subsequent dose cannot be given for a preset period, the 'lockout period'.
- Typical settings for an adult using morphine (Table 8.4) delivered by a PCA device might be:
  - bolus dose: 1 mg;
  - lockout interval: 5 minutes.

- PCA devices record attempts made by the patient to access analgesia, allowing the dose to be adjusted to meet their requirements.

Effective PCA requires the following.

- The patient to be briefed by the anaesthetist and/or nursing staff preoperatively and, if possible, be shown the device to be used.
- A loading dose of analgesic, usually intravenously before starting. Failure to do this will result in the patient being unable to get sufficient analgesia from the PCA device and the system will fail.

Table 8.4 Morphine preparations.

Oral	Immediate-release (IR) tablets or liquid:
	• Absorption and effect within minutes
	• Usual adult dose 20 mg 2 hourly prn
	• Less in elderly, more if opioid tolerant
	• Providing the gut is working, useful even after major surgery
	• Usually used for acute pain where the opioid requirement is unknown or changing rapidly
	Modified-release (MR) tablets, capsules or granules:
	• Dose released over either 12 or 24 hours
	• Avoids frequent dosing with IR preparations
	• Used in 10 mg or 20 mg doses in a reducing regimen in enhanced recovery
	• Useful when opioid requirement is prolonged and also for gradually weaning down the dose at the end of treatment
	The two formulations are usually used together to provide a steady background level of analgesa (MR) with additional breakthrough doses (IR) as required
	It is important that everybody understands the difference between MR and IR forms of morphine
IV	Morphine 10 or 20 mg diluted to 1 mg/mL with 0.9% sodium chloride can be given:
	• in increments initially of 1–3 mg at 3-minute intervals; effective dose may range from 1 to 50 mg or more (the latter in opioid-tolerant patients)
	• via patient-controlled analgesia device (see text)
	• as a continuous infusion. Useful where patient cooperation is limited, e.g. in elderly patients or ITU. Problems occur in predicting the correct infusion rate, given the variability of dose requirement between patients. Very close supervision is required to avoid underinfusion (pain) or overinfusion (toxicity). This method can be used to replace high doses of oral opioids during the perioperative period
	The intravenous dose of morphine is about one-third of the oral dose
IM	A predetermined dose (e.g. morphine 10 mg) at fixed minimum intervals, e.g. hourly
	• Delayed and variable rate of effect
	• Precise titration is difficult with repeated cycles of pain and relief
	• Does not require complex equipment or a cooperative patient
	• Although widely available, gradually being replaced by the above

ITU, intensive therapy unit.

- A dedicated IV cannula or non-return valve on an IV infusion to prevent accumulation of the drug and failure of analgesia.
- Observation and recording of the patient's pain score, sedation score and respiratory rate is essential to ensure success. Any patient with a respiratory rate less than 8 breaths/minute and a sedation score of 2 or 3 requires immediate intervention:
  - stop the PCA;
  - give oxygen via a mask;
  - call for assistance;
  - consider giving naloxone (see earlier in this chapter);
  - if the patient is apnoeic, commence ventilation using a self-inflating bag-valve-mask device.

Advantages of PCA

- Greater flexibility; analgesia matched to the patient's perception of the pain.
- Reduced workload for the nursing staff.
- Elimination of painful intramuscular (IM) injections.
- Drug given IV with greater certainty of adequate plasma levels.

Disadvantages of PCA

- Equipment is expensive to purchase and maintain.
- It requires patient comprehension of the system.
- Patient must be physically able to trigger the device.
- The elderly are often reluctant to use a PCA device.
- The potential for overdose if the device is incorrectly programmed.

As pain subsides, the PCA can be discontinued and oral analgesics can be used. The first oral dose should be given 1 hour prior to discontinuing PCA, to ensure continuity of analgesia.

Regional analgesic techniques (Figure 8.7)

- *Peripheral nerve blocks*: used mainly for pain relief after upper or lower limb surgery. A single injection of local anaesthetic, usually bupivacaine, results in 6–12 hours of pain relief. An infusion of local anaesthetic via a catheter inserted close to the nerve may enable the block to be continued for several days. An alternative and effective form of analgesia must be prescribed for when the local anaesthetic is discontinued to prevent the patient being in severe pain.

- *Transversus abdominis plane (TAP) block (see Chapter 6)*: infusion of local anaesthetic via a catheter placed in the plane between the transversus abdominis and internal oblique muscles to anaesthetize the nerves supplying the skin and muscles of the anterior abdominal wall (and parietal peritoneum).
- *Epidural analgesia (see Chapter 6)*: infusions of a local anaesthetic into the epidural space, either alone or in combination with opioids, act on the transiting nerve roots and the dorsal horn of the spinal cord, respectively. The aim is to 'block' all of the nerve roots that carry sensory nerves from the area of tissue injury to provide dramatic relief of postoperative pain. It is essential that patients who are offered an epidural receive an explanation from the anaesthetist at the preoperative visit of what to expect postoperatively, in particular altered sensation, weakness of the lower limbs and the potential need for a urinary catheter [8.4]. The epidural is often sited preoperatively and used intraoperatively as part of the anaesthetic technique. For upper abdominal surgery, an epidural in the midthoracic region (T6–7) is used, while a hip operation would need a lumbar epidural (L1–2).

Different combinations of local anaesthetic and opioid infusion have been used successfully. Ideally, the concentration of local anaesthetic should selectively block sensory nerves, with relative sparing of motor nerves. The choice and dose of opioid should be such that the drug passes through the dura into the CSF in sufficient quantities to block the opioid receptors in the spinal cord but not spread cranially to cause respiratory depression, for example levobupivacaine 0.125% plus fentanyl 2–4 µg/mL. Epidural infusions can be used to maintain analgesia for several days. Opioid side-effects are less common and less severe than when given systemically as the dose is much less.

There are a number of important points to bear in mind when using epidural analgesia.

- The infusion rate and the site of the catheter determine the spread of the solution. The greater the anatomical area, i.e. increasing number of dermatomes requiring blockade, the greater the rate of infusion required, approximately 1–2 mL/hour per dermatome.
- The efficacy of the infusion must be monitored in a similar manner as for PCA.
- If analgesia is inadequate, a 'top-up' of 5–10 mL of solution may be necessary.

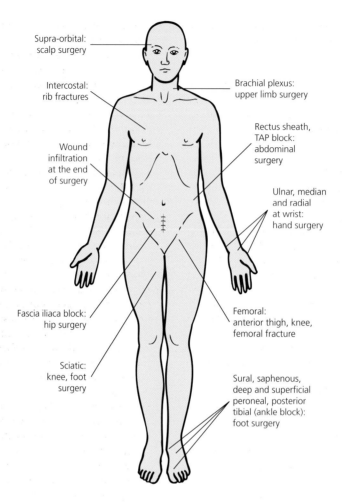

Supra-orbital:
scalp surgery

Intercostal:
rib fractures

Brachial plexus:
upper limb surgery

Wound
infiltration
at the end
of surgery

Rectus sheath,
TAP block:
abdominal
surgery

Ulnar, median
and radial
at wrist:
hand surgery

Fascia iliaca block:
hip surgery

Femoral:
anterior thigh, knee,
femoral fracture

Sciatic:
knee, foot
surgery

Sural, saphenous,
deep and superficial
peroneal, posterior
tibial (ankle block):
foot surgery

Figure 8.7 Some commonly used nerve blocks. TAP, transversus abdominis plane.

- Observations of the patient's vital signs should then be made on a regular basis according to local protocol.
- In patients over the age of 60 years, the concentration of opioid is often halved.

Management of complications during postoperative epidural analgesia

The complications arising as a result of the use of local anaesthetics are the same as when they are used intraoperatively, and are covered in Chapter 6. All patients having epidural analgesia require regular monitoring and documentation of:

- heart rate and blood pressure;
- respiratory rate and peripheral oxygen saturations;

- urine output;
- pain scores at rest and on movement;
- lower limb motor function;
- conscious level, usually assessed using the Glasgow Coma Scale (GCS) score.

As a general rule, any complications related to an epidural should be discussed with an anaesthetist or the hospital's acute pain team. There are a number of complications that may present whilst a patient is receiving epidural analgesia or after it has been stopped.

- *Hypotension*: due to block of the sympathetic nerves:
  - block of T2–L2 results in vasodilatation, a drop in systemic vascular resistance and hypotension;
  - block of the thoracic nerve roots above T5 also reduces heart rate and contractility;

- patients with additional fluid losses, for example haemorrhage, are particularly vulnerable to severe hypotension;
- the legs can be raised to counteract the vasodilatation, the equivalent to a 500 mL fluid challenge;
- a fluid bolus, for example 500 mL Hartmann's, should be given immediately; a vasopressor can also be given, for example ephedrine 3–6 mg IV. An infusion of a vasopressor can also be used which prevents the need for repeated and excessive fluid boluses;
- a bradycardia with 'adverse features' should be treated with atropine 500 µg IV;
- the extent of the block should be checked, the epidural infusion may need to be stopped or the rate reduced, and an anaesthetist called urgently to plan further management;
- the patient may need admission to a critical care area for close monitoring as the effect of the epidural anaesthetic already given may last for several hours.

- *Respiratory depression*: due to systemic absorption of the opioid or secondary to block of the thoracic nerve roots:
  - highly lipid-soluble opioids (diamorphine, fentanyl) are rapidly taken up by the spinal cord, limiting their spread and systemic absorption, and respiratory depression tends to occur early; less soluble opioids (morphine) are taken up slowly, and respiratory depression tends to occur later;
  - motor block above T4 will paralyse the intercostal muscles, impairing ventilation;
  - evaluation of the block height and risk factors for opioid sensitivity will help determine which is most likely;
  - in either case, stop the epidural infusion, at least temporarily;
  - if opioid narcosis is suspected, give 100–200 µg of naloxone IV;
  - support ventilation if necessary;
  - seek expert help.

- *Urinary retention*: due to both the loss of the sensation of a full bladder and the direct effect of opioids on the sphincter muscles:
  - commoner in males, particularly if there are already symptoms of prostatism;
  - urinary retention usually results in complete anuria, and the bladder may be palpable in the suprapubic area of the abdomen;
  - oliguria is more likely to be due to hypotension or hypovolaemia, or other intra-abdominal pathology, and needs appropriate management depending on the cause;
  - it may be prevented by routine monitoring of urine output in all postoperative patients;
  - it may require short-term catheterization.

- *Motor block (leg weakness)*: this is commonest when concentrated local anaesthetic solutions (0.25% or 0.5% levo-bupivacaine) are used; it is less frequent with low concentrations (0.1–0.125% levo-bupivacaine):
  - it may lead to pressure ulcers on the patient's heels or sacrum due to lack of movement, or falls whilst mobilizing;
  - the infusion should be stopped and the anaesthetic/pain team informed;
  - it may be prevented by regular observation of effects of the epidural and correct adjustment of infusion rate.

- *Inadequate analgesia*: this is usually a consequence of inadequate spread of the local anaesthetic solution to all nerve roots:
  - a bolus dose of local anaesthetic may be required and the rate of infusion may need to be increased – this should be done by an anaesthetist familiar with epidural analgesia;
  - there may be pain from sites not covered by the epidural, for example pain referred to the shoulder due to diaphragmatic irritation:
    - it may require alternative systemic analgesia;
    - systemic opioids should not be given if the epidural solution contains an opioid.

- *Pruritus*: this can be severe and frequently localized to the nose; it may respond to antihistamines, atropine or naloxone.

- *Headache*: occurs in 0.5–1% of epidurals, due to puncture of the dura by the needle (or catheter) and subsequent CSF leak. This is often referred to as a 'postdural puncture headache' (PDPH):
  - it may or may not be recognized at the time of performing the epidural;
  - it typically develops 24–48 hours after epidural insertion and is worse on sitting or standing and better on lying down;
  - an anaesthetist should be informed, who can assess the patient and discuss appropriate management, possibly an epidural 'blood patch';
  - many headaches respond well to simple measures such as paracetamol, NSAIDs and good fluid intake.

Worsening or severe leg weakness is not a normal feature of epidural analgesia and needs investigating urgently. Possible causes include the following.

- Intrathecal migration of the epidural catheter – the local anaesthetic is then delivered intrathecally causing an extensive spinal anaesthesia.
- Epidural haematoma – the risk is greater in patients on anticoagulants or antiplatelet drugs, those with a coagulopathy or thrombocytopenia.
- Epidural abscess – an infection introduced via the catheter, which is commoner with prolonged use of an epidural:
  - haematomas and abscesses can produce symptoms after the catheter has been removed;
  - patients complain typically of increasing back pain;
  - this may be delayed so that the connection to the surgery and epidural may be missed (up to several weeks later in the case of abscess);
  - if an epidural haematoma or abscess is suspected, the investigation of choice is urgent magnetic resonance (MR) scanning.
- Damage to nerves or the spinal cord during insertion of the needle and systemic toxicity of the local anaesthetic. These are both unusual complications.

 KEY POINT

- Any patient with an epidural who develops increasing motor blockade in the absence of excessive anaesthetic doses needs urgent investigation by a senior anaesthetist.

Intrathecal (spinal) analgesia

Spinal anaesthesia is of insufficient duration to provide postoperative pain relief. However, if a small dose of opioid, for example diamorphine 250–500 μg, is injected along with the local anaesthetic, this may provide 12–24 hours of analgesia. Complications are the same as those due to opioids given epidurally and are managed in the same way.

Other techniques

Entonox is a mixture of nitrous oxide (50%) and oxygen (50%). It is a weak analgesic with sedative properties and is useful for short-term analgesia for painful procedures, such as change of dressings. It should be avoided in patients with a pneumothorax because the nitrous oxide may diffuse into the gas-filled space, increasing the volume.

Difficult pain problems

Patients who show evidence of regular opioid use preoperatively, such as drug addicts, cancer and chronic pain patients and those patients with a previous bad pain experience, may pose a particular problem postoperatively. They are best managed if they are identified at the preoperative assessment and a team approach is used that will include:

- liaison with the acute pain team to inform them of the patient's admission;
- discussion with the anaesthetist, and surgical and nursing staff to plan perioperative care, to:
  - ensure any current opioid medication is continued on admission to prevent withdrawal;
  - understand that much larger doses of opioids than normal may be required;
  - explain that toxicity from high doses of opioid is very unlikely;
  - reassure that addiction is not a concern;
- discussion with the patient to explain:
  - types and effectiveness of analgesic regimes available postoperatively;
  - that analgesia may not be 100% effective;
  - that long-term continuation may be necessary;
  - potential side-effects, especially if regional analgesia planned;
- plan regular reviews during the postoperative period;
- early use of alternative analgesics, e.g. ketamine infusion, magnesium, dexamethasone;
- coordination of care.

Enhanced recovery

This process was first described in the 1990s in Copenhagen, with the aim of improving the speed and quality of patients' recovery after surgery and reducing their length of stay in hospital, and it has been in increasing use in the United Kingdom since around 2000 [8.5]. There are a number of key elements of an enhanced recovery programme.

1 Preoperative assessment and care planning:
  - full physical and psychological assessment;
  - anaesthesia planning – consultation with anaesthetist, use of regional techniques;

- discussion of immediate postoperative course – pain, analgesia, catheters, mobilization;
- physical optimization – diet, exercise, weight loss, physiotherapy (also called prehabilitation), good control of co-morbidities, e.g. hypertension, diabetes;
- discharge planning – length of stay, home equipment, support services, e.g. physiotherapy, GP involvement;
- complete consent process.

2 Operative management:
- use of minimally invasive surgical techniques, e.g. laparoscopic techniques;
- controlled IV fluid therapy – use of ultrasound/echo to guide volume replacement;
- use of short-acting anaesthetic drugs;
- selective use of regional anaesthesia, taking care not to prevent early mobilisation, e.g. low-dose epidural, spinal opioids, TAP blocks, paravertebral blocks;
- temperature control;
- multimodal antiemetic therapy where necessary;
- prophylactic antibiotics;
- deep venous thrombosis (DVT) prophylaxis.

3 Immediate postoperative management:
- multimodal analgesia, low-dose epidural infusions;
- avoid systemic opioids where possible;
- early mobilization and physiotherapy;
- prophylactic use of antiemetics;
- minimize use of IV fluids, nasogastric tubes, urinary catheters;
- early, normal diet.

4 Late postoperative management:
- regular analgesia – use paracetamol, NSAIDs, avoid opioids when possible;
- mobilization in accordance with preoperative planning;
- diet.

5 Discharge:
- ensure all facilities are in place before discharge – use a checklist;
- liaison with support services, e.g. GP, community nursing;
- ensure follow-up processes in place, agreed and understood;
- audit complication, readmission rate, patient satisfaction.

If correctly conducted, enhanced recovery programmes result in reduced length of hospital stay, fewer postoperative complications, reduced readmissions and improved patient outcomes. However, success requires appropriate training of staff, resources, specific care plans and engagement with the patients, their families and care in the community [8.6].

FURTHER INFORMATION

Bay I, Nunn JF, Prys Roberts C. Factors affecting arterial PO_2 during recovery from general anaesthesia. *British Journal of Anaesthesia* 1968; **40**: 398–407.

Gan TJ, Meyer T, Apfel CC, *et al*. Consensus guidelines for managing postoperative nausea and vomiting. *Anesthesia and Analgesia* 2003; **97**: 62–71.

Thomson AJ, Webb DJ, Maxwell SRJ, Grant IS. Oxygen therapy in acute medical care. *British Medical Journal* 2002; **324**: 1406–1407.

West JB. *Respiratory Physiology: The Essentials*, 9th edn. Baltimore: Williams & Wilkins, 2011.

[8.1] www.aagbi.org/sites/default/files/immediate_postanaesthesia_recovery_2013.pdf
Immediate Post-anaesthesia recovery. AAGBI, 2013.

[8.2] www.brit-thoracic.org.uk/document-library/clinical-information/oxygen/emergency-oxygen-use-in-adult-patients-guideline/emergency-oxygen-use-in-adult-patients-guideline/
British Thoracic Society guidelines for the use of oxygen in adult patients. To be updated in 2016.

[8.3] www.medicine.ox.ac.uk/bandolier/booth/painpag/index2.html
The Oxford Pain site. Brilliant for the latest evidence-based information on all aspects of acute pain.

[8.4] www.rcoa.ac.uk/system/files/FPM-EpAnalg2010_1.pdf
Best practice in the management of epidural analgesia in the hospital setting. Royal College of Anaesthetists, 2010.

[8.5] www.erassociety.org
Enhanced recovery after surgery web site. Up-to-date information on recovery after surgery.

[8.6] www.reducinglengthofstay.org.uk/doc/isog_report.pdf
Improving Surgical Outcome Group. Interesting report on how outcomes after major surgery can be improved.

9

Perioperative medical emergencies: recognition and management

Clinical Anaesthesia: Lecture Notes, Fifth Edition. Matthew Gwinnutt
and Carl Gwinnutt.
© 2017 John Wiley & Sons, Ltd. Published 2017 by John Wiley & Sons, Ltd.
Companion website: www.lecturenoteseries.com/anaesthesia

Section 1: Recognition and assessment

The focus of this chapter is on how to recognize and initially manage acute problems commonly encountered on general hospital wards and how to refer such patients effectively to senior colleagues if there is not a prompt improvement in the patient's condition in response to initial management. All too often, misinterpretation of the clinical picture may lead either to a lack of action or to treatment being commenced that is inappropriate. A classic anecdotal example is the elderly postoperative patient who is breathless, hypotensive and oliguric and has crackles on auscultation of the chest. Acute heart failure is diagnosed and a large dose of an intravenous (IV) diuretic is given. The correct diagnosis may in fact be pneumonia, sepsis and pre-renal failure secondary to hypovolaemia and hypotension. Although the intravenous diuretic may initially increase urine output, ultimately it will exacerbate the dehydration and pre-renal failure, and may even precipitate acute cardiovascular collapse.

The immediate aim is to identify dysfunction in one or more organ systems and initiate appropriate treatment to prevent further deterioration before frank organ system failure supervenes. Once this has been achieved, appropriate investigations will help to make a clinical diagnosis of the cause of the patient's illness. Even if this is not possible, early referral for higher level care (for example, transfer to a high-dependency unit (HDU) or intensive therapy unit (ITU)) will improve the patient's prognosis. Attending a moribund patient on the ward in extremis or, even worse, in cardiac arrest should generally be seen as a failure of previous management. Mortality increases with illness severity and the outcome after cardiac arrest in hospitalized patients is extremely poor, with less than 20% patients surviving to hospital discharge.

Although there are exceptions (such as acute massive pulmonary embolism in a postoperative patient or ventricular fibrillation cardiac arrest post myocardial infarction), critical life-threatening illness tends to develop gradually over hours or days. Although the presenting illness often involves only one organ system, the lack of appropriate management may result in multiple organ systems becoming involved and ultimately one or more organs may fail as the patient's physiological compensatory mechanisms become exhausted.

In an ideal world, the doctor attending an acutely ill patient would be a senior, experienced clinician who would expertly make a rapid assessment of the patient, initiate emergency treatment, carry out a more detailed assessment, order appropriate investigations and finally arrive at a likely clinical diagnosis and initiate definitive treatment. In the real world this is usually not the case. Routine procedure for the ward nurse concerned about a patient's condition will be to contact the most junior member of the medical team, often a Foundation Year One doctor. The reason for the call may have been that the patient's Early Warning Score (EWS – see later) has exceeded a trigger threshold. However, the nurse may also be more specific in stating that she is worried about the patient's breathing, low blood pressure, low urine output, and so on. The inexperienced clinician will need to rely on a systematic process of clinical assessment to identify which organ systems are dysfunctional or failing, what the likely diagnosis is (or differential diagnoses are) and therefore what initial management is most appropriate [9.1].

Although ultimately there is no substitute for experience, a diverse range of courses is available, which aim to 'short-circuit' the knowledge and experience gap. These courses provide intensive, often didactic teaching by faculties of experienced multidisciplinary clinicians, including doctors and nurses from different specialties. Examples include the following.

- *Acute Life-threatening Event Recognition and Treatment (ALERT)*: the recognition and management of patients in the early stages of developing critical illness.
- *Acute Illness Management (AIM)*: the recognition and management of patients in the early stages of developing critical illness.
- *Care of the Critically Ill Surgical Patient (CCrISP)*: the management of critically ill surgical patients.
- *Advanced Life Support (ALS)*: the prevention and management of cardiorespiratory arrest.
- *European Trauma Course (ETC)*: the management of major life-threatening trauma.
- *European Paediatric Life Support (EPLS)*: the early recognition of the child in respiratory or circulatory failure.
- *Advanced Paediatric Life Support (APLS)*: the recognition and management of the sick child.

Attendance at an ALS course is mandatory for Foundation doctors (as is successfully passing the course!) and attending at least one of the courses aimed at recognizing and managing acutely ill patients cannot be recommended highly enough.

Clinical scoring systems (track and trigger systems)

In order to treat acute illness or the deterioration in a patient's condition, it first has to be recognized, often by the ward nurse in response to routine clinical observations. In the 1990s, formal clinical scoring systems, often termed Early Warning Scoring systems (EWS), were introduced to facilitate the process of assessing illness severity, 'flagging up' patients for urgent medical assessment and monitoring response to treatment. In 2007, the National Institute for Health and Clinical (now Care) Excellence (NICE) published its guidance on the recognition and response to acute illness in adults [9.2]. This recommended that 'Physiological track and trigger systems should be used to monitor all adult patients in acute hospital settings'.

All EWS systems are based on the premise that acute physiological deterioration precedes the development of life-threatening acute illness and cardiorespiratory arrest. Simple observations relating to the physiological and clinical status of the patient that can be performed at the bedside on a general ward are recorded and scores are allocated for each observation based on reference to a scoring table. In 2012,

the Royal College of Physicians published a National Early Warning Score (NEWS) [9.3]. This was an attempt to try and standardize the assessment process and link the scoring system to clearly defined levels of action that would ensure an effective clinical response at all times (Figure 9.1).

The NEWS cannot cover every patient, in every situation, and there may be times when an acceptance of different 'normal values' may be appropriate.

In some settings, patients will have an impaired level of consciousness as a consequence of sedation, e.g. following surgical procedures. Thus, the assessment of conscious level and the necessity to escalate care should be considered in context of the appropriateness of the conscious level in relation to recent sedation.

For patients with known hypercapnic respiratory failure due to chronic obstructive pulmonary disease (COPD), the British Thoracic Society target saturations of 88–92% should be used [8.2]. These patients will still 'score' if their oxygen saturations are below 92% unless the score is 'reset' by a competent clinical decision-maker and patient-specific target oxygen saturations are prescribed and documented on the chart and in the clinical notes. All supplemental oxygen, when given, must be prescribed.

National Early Warning Score (NEWS)*

PHYSIOLOGICAL PARAMETERS	3	2	1	0	1	2	3
Respiration rate	≤8		9–11	12–20		21–24	≥25
Oxygen saturations	≤91	92–93	94–95	≥96			
Any supplemental oxygen		Yes		No			
Temperature	≤35.0		35.1–36.0	36.1–38.0	38.1–39.0	≥39.1	
Systolic BP	≤90	91–100	101–110	111–219			≥220
Heart rate	≤40		41–50	51–90	91–110	111–130	≥131
Level of consciousness				A			V, P, or U

*The NEWS initiative flowed from the Royal College of Physicians' NEWS Development and Implementation Group (NEWSDIG) report, and was jointly developed and funded in collaboration with the Royal College of Physicians, Royal College of Nursing, National Outreach Forum and NHS Training for Innovation

Royal College of Physicians

NHS *Training for Innovation*

© Royal College of Physicians 2012

Figure 9.1 The National Early Warning Scoring system. Source: Royal College of Physicians, 2012.

To facilitate standardization and a national unified approach, a colour-coded clinical chart has been developed. Ideally, this would be used across the NHS to record routine clinical data and track a patient's clinical condition. This tracking system will alert the clinical team to any untoward clinical deterioration and also clinical recovery. The individual scores derived from each variable are aggregated and trigger thresholds are set that mandate action dependent on whether the aggregated score is low, medium or high:

- *low score (NEWS 1–4)*: assessment by a competent nurse to decide if a change to the frequency of monitoring or escalation of clinical care is required;
- *medium score (NEWS 5–6 or any single 'red' [3] score)*: urgent review by a clinician trained and competent in the assessment and management of acute illness. Consideration must be given to whether escalation to a team with critical care skills is required;
- *high score (NEWS ≥7)*: emergency assessment by a member of a critical care outreach team. Transfer will also usually be required to a higher level of care.

The main advantages of such scoring systems are:

- simplicity, with the need for only the basic monitoring equipment, normally present on any acute hospital ward;
- reproducibility between different observers;
- staff require a minimum of training;
- their applicability to trainee doctors, nurses (both qualified and student) and other health professionals.

Clinical scoring systems are undoubtedly useful but they cannot be relied upon to the exclusion of sound clinical judgement. They fail to identify some patients who are at risk (false negatives, low sensitivity) and identify other patients as being at risk when they are not (false positives, low specificity).

Critical care outreach teams

Outreach teams (sometimes called medical emergency teams (METs)) have been established in many hospitals to either respond to a patient with a high EWS or to assist the medical team to manage a patient who is not responding to treatment. Outreach teams are usually multidisciplinary, with their precise make-up varying from hospital to hospital. The team leader should be trained in the management of critically ill patients and ideally be either an experienced critical care doctor or critical care nurse practitioner.

Table 9.1 Aims of the outreach team.

- Early identification of patients with actual or potential critical illness
- Appropriate early intervention, which may prevent deterioration and avert the need for admission to HDU or ITU
- Liaison with the HDU and ITU
- Facilitate early admission to HDU and ITU when necessary
- Identification of patients for whom HDU or ITU care is deemed inappropriate
- Appropriate early designation of patients as 'do not attempt resuscitation' in the event of cardiorespiratory arrest (DNACPR order)
- To assist ward nurses in the management of patients with actual or potential critical illness
- Education and training of trainee doctors, nurses and medical students
- Promote continuity of care following step-down of patients to the ward from HDU and ITU

HDU, high-dependency unit; ITU, intensive therapy unit.

Table 9.2 SBAR and RSVP communication tools.

S – Situation	R – Reason for calling
B – Background	S – Story
A – Assessment (plus any NEWS)	V – Vital signs (plus any NEWS)
R – Recommendation	P – Plan

The aims of the outreach team are summarized in Table 9.1.

Receiving a call

When called to assess an acutely ill patient, you may not have seen him/her previously and may have no prior knowledge of his/her medical history. Therefore, when answering a call to assess a sick patient, it is very helpful to be given information in a structured manner, so that you can be thinking about possible causes and treatment as you make your way to the ward. The two most commonly used structures for conveying information are 'Situation, Background, Assessment, Response' (SBAR) and 'Reason, Story, Vital signs, Plan' (RSVP) [9.4]. These are summarized in Table 9.2.

Principles of assessment

When assessing and managing acutely ill patients, irrespective of the severity of their conditions, the initial aim must be to make the patient safe rather than to determine a precise diagnosis. Many clinical crises can initially be managed by prompt recognition and correction of a modest number of common abnormalities using simple therapies (for example, oxygen and fluids).

It is logical for all members of the healthcare team to use the same systematic approach to assess and treat the 'at risk' or acutely ill patient incorporating the following:

- primary assessment and resuscitation using the 'ABCDE' approach;
- start simple bedside monitoring;
- once immediate life-threatening conditions have been treated, secondary assessment of the patient using all available information – history, examination, investigations;
- analysis of all the information available and making a diagnosis or a list of differential diagnoses;
- a definitive management or care plan, including referral to a senior colleague if you have any doubts about your ability to manage the situation safely;
- good record keeping.

 KEY POINTS

- The aim of initial interventions is to keep the patient alive and produce some clinical improvement, so that definitive treatment may be initiated.
- Always correct life-threatening abnormalities before moving on to the next stage of the assessment.
- Resuscitation measures (oxygen, fluids, etc.) often take a few minutes to have an effect.
- Call for help early. At every stage of the patient assessment, consider 'do I need help?'

Once immediately life-threatening conditions have been identified and treated following your primary assessment, undertake a full secondary assessment. Reassess the patient regularly and after every intervention to determine the impact of treatment and to detect any deterioration. Do not try to do everything yourself; use all members of the multidisciplinary team – they are there to help you. Use a structured approach as described above to ensure all relevant information is passed on. There may be several interventions happening at the same time, particularly if the patient is in a peri-arrest situation; always ensure your own safety and that of the patient:

- take note of environmental hazards such as electricity and fluid spillage;
- dispose of needles and other sharps into 'sharps bins';
- protect yourself by taking universal precautions – aprons, gloves and masks will reduce the risk of contamination from secretions, blood and so forth.

Infection prevention and control has an important impact on patient outcome; therefore, despite all the pressures:

- always wash your hands before and after patient contact;
- adopt an aseptic no-touch technique (ANTT) for invasive procedures.

Initial approach to the patient

Ask the patient a simple question, such as 'How are you?' A normal verbal response immediately informs you that the patient:

- has a patent airway;
- is breathing;
- has brain perfusion with oxygenated blood.

If the patient can only speak in short sentences, suspect severe respiratory distress. Failure to respond to the question is likely to suggest serious illness and you should immediately assess the patient for signs of life whilst keeping the airway open. If the patient has no signs of life, follow the current guidelines for in-hospital resuscitation (see later).

The next step is to commence an ABCDE assessment of the patient. While you are doing this, ask an assistant to attach the following as soon as possible:

- pulse oximeter;
- electrocardiogram (ECG) monitor;
- non-invasive blood pressure monitor.

The ABCDE system is as follows.

- A is for AIRWAY
- B is for BREATHING
- C is for CIRCULATION

- D is for DISABILITY (central nervous system (CNS) function)
- E is for EXPOSURE (permitting full patient examination)

The assessment and consequent actions are prioritized in this order because, generally, airway obstruction kills faster than breathing disorders, which in turn kill faster than blood loss or cardiac dysfunction. Each part of the assessment system follows a similar pattern – the simultaneous identification and treatment of potentially life-threatening conditions.

Most abnormalities will be detected using simple clinical examination techniques based on a look-listen-feel approach. The order of the components of the look-listen-feel approach will vary depending on the body system being examined.

Primary assessment and resuscitation

Airway assessment (A)

The aim is to identify and treat airway obstruction if present. Always treat airway obstruction as a medical emergency and obtain expert help immediately. Untreated, it leads to a lowered PaO_2, and risks hypoxic damage to the vital organs (brain, kidneys and heart) and will cause cardiac arrest and death. In a critically ill patient, airway obstruction is frequently due to a depressed conscious level but there are other causes (Table 9.3).

 KEY POINTS

- Impaired conscious level, for example due to cerebral hypoxia, drugs or acute brain injury, is the commonest cause of airway obstruction on general hospital wards.
- Noisy breathing always indicates obstruction; silence may mean apnoea.

Look, listen and feel for the signs of airway obstruction. This is best accomplished by positioning your ear close to the patient's nose and mouth whilst looking down across the chest.

Look for chest movement

- Paradoxical chest and abdominal movements ('see-saw' respirations).

Table 9.3 Causes of acute upper airway obstruction.

- Depressed conscious level
- Secretions, blood, vomit
- Foreign body
- Upper airway swelling
- Upper airway tumour
- External compression of the airway
- Blocked tracheostomy
- Trauma

Table 9.4 Characteristics of airway noises to assist in localizing the level of airway obstruction.

Sound	Cause
• Gurgling	• Liquid in the mouth or upper airway
• Snoring	• Partial obstruction of the pharynx, usually by the tongue
• Crowing	• Laryngeal spasm
• Inspiratory stridor	• Obstruction above or at the level of the larynx
• Expiratory wheeze	• Airway collapse during expiration (e.g. asthma)
• Rattling	• Secretions in the airways

- Use of the accessory muscles of respiration (for example, sternomastoid and muscles of the neck, back and shoulder girdle).

NOTE: central cyanosis is a late sign of airway obstruction.

Listen for sounds of air movement and any associated abnormal noises

- Complete airway obstruction is silent.
- Partial airway obstruction is noisy.
- Silence indicates either complete airway obstruction in the presence of the patient's obvious efforts to breathe or apnoea (respiratory arrest).

Certain noises assist in localizing the level of the obstruction (Table 9.4).

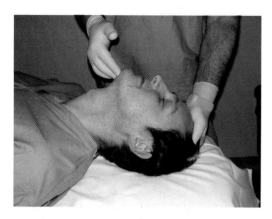

Figure 9.2 Head tilt and chin lift.

Feel for expired air

- Place your hand or side of face immediately in front of the patient's mouth. This will help confirm the presence or absence of airflow and give an indication of the tidal volume.

If there are signs of obstruction, call for expert help immediately and rapidly move to using simple methods of airway clearance: a visual inspection for evidence of obvious upper airway obstruction due to a foreign body (for example, blood, secretions, food bolus, vomit) and careful airway suction only as far as you can see using a rigid wide-bore suction catheter (for example, Yankauer). Perform a head tilt and chin lift (Figure 9.2) and insertion of an oropharyngeal or nasopharyngeal airway (see Chapter 5). If these measures fail, tracheal intubation may be required, but should only be attempted by experienced staff. In most situations, intubation will require the use of a hypnotic and neuromuscular blocking drugs and an anaesthetist.

Once you are certain that the patient has a satisfactory airway, give oxygen initially at high flow (15 L/minute) using a mask with an oxygen reservoir (see Figure 8.4), and move on rapidly to assess breathing. This applies to all patients who are breathless or who exhibit other signs of acute illness, including patients with COPD. Hypoxia kills quickly; hypercapnia kills much more slowly. Reassess the patient and once stable, titrate the inspired oxygen to produce an acceptable SpO_2 or PaO_2 (see later).

Assess breathing (B)

The aim is to assess adequacy of breathing and to diagnose and treat immediately life-threatening conditions: severe bronchospasm, severe pneumonia,

Table 9.5 Causes of breathing problems.

Primary lung dysfunction	Secondary causes
Acute	**Respiratory**
• Acute asthma	• Airway obstruction
• Pneumonia	• ARDS
• Pneumothorax	• Aspiration
• Acute exacerbation of COPD	**Cardiovascular**
• Exhaustion	• Heart failure
• Haemothorax	• Pulmonary embolism
• Pulmonary contusion	• Cardiac tamponade
Chronic	**Neuromuscular problems**
• Emphysema	• Guillain–Barré syndrome
• Pulmonary fibrosis	• Myasthenia gravis
• Tumours	• High spinal cord injury
• Bronchiectasis	• Exhaustion
• Cystic fibrosis	**CNS depression**
• Tuberculosis	• Drugs
• Diffuse parenchymal lung disease	• Head injury
	• Meningitis/encephalitis
	• Cerebral haemorrhage
	• Cerebral tumour
	• Cerebral hypoxia
	Diaphragmatic splinting
	• Morbidly obese patients
	• Abdominal pain
	• Abdominal distension

ARDS, acute respiratory distress syndrome; CNS, central nervous system; COPD, chronic obstructive pulmonary disease.

acute exacerbation of COPD, acute pulmonary oedema and tension pneumothorax. If untreated, inadequate breathing will lead to hypoxaemia and may also cause hypercapnia (see Figures 8.1, 8.2), which can eventually lead to unconsciousness. There are many causes of disordered or inadequate breathing (Table 9.5). Use the look-listen-feel approach.

Look for the signs of abnormal breathing

- Use of the accessory muscles of respiration, tracheal tug, abdominal breathing, sweating, central cyanosis.

- Normal is between 12 and 20 breaths/minute. A rapid rate is an early sign of severe acute illness and should be regarded as a warning that the patient may suddenly deteriorate; an abnormally low rate suggests a CNS problem.
- The depth of each breath.
- The pattern (rhythm) of breathing.
- The symmetry of movement of the two sides of the chest.

Also look for:

- chest deformity, as this may impair the ability to breathe normally;
- raised jugular venous pressure (JVP) (which may signify acute severe asthma or a tension pneumothorax);
- chest drains – are they patent, below the level of the chest and swinging/draining?
- abdominal distension, as this may exacerbate respiratory distress by limiting diaphragmatic movement.

Listen for signs of respiratory disease

- Place your ear close to the patient's face if necessary. Rattling or gurgling airway noises indicate the presence of airway secretions, often due to the inability of the patient to cough sufficiently or to take a deep breath. Inspiratory noisy breathing (stridor) suggests partial, but significant, airway obstruction.
- Auscultate the chest, placing the stethoscope in all areas of the chest, both front and back, and assess the quality of the breath sounds:
  o high-pitched expiratory noisy breathing (wheeze) suggests bronchospasm;
  o bronchial breathing suggests lung consolidation;
  o absent or reduced sounds suggest the presence of a pneumothorax or pleural effusion;
  o crackles – if fine, they suggest pulmonary oedema or pulmonary fibrosis; coarse crackles suggest retained secretions.

Feel the chest

Check the following.

- The position of the trachea in the suprasternal notch. Deviation to one side indicates mediastinal shift (for example, tension pneumothorax or massive pleural effusion).
- Equality of expansion – reduced on the side of a pneumothorax or pleural effusion.
- Surgical emphysema or crepitus – assume that this indicates a pneumothorax until proven otherwise.

- Percussion: hyperresonance suggests a pneumothorax; dullness suggests consolidation or pleural fluid.

Attach a pulse oximeter to the patient as soon as possible; this provides invaluable information on the net result of the patient's respiratory effort in oxygenating blood as it flows through the lungs. In most patients, the target SpO_2 should be 94–98%. Initially, give high-flow oxygen at 15 L/minute using a mask with attached reservoir bag; the inspired oxygen may be reduced later according to the patient's response. Some patients suffering from **severe** COPD (type II respiratory failure, chronic hypoxaemia and hypercapnia) may develop increasing hypercapnia if given a high inspired oxygen concentration. This is mainly a consequence of a loss of hypoxic pulmonary vasoconstriction (which worsens V/Q matching) and changes in the CO_2 buffering capacity of the blood. In these patients, careful titration of the inspired oxygen concentration should allow improvement in the PaO_2 without causing a significant increase in $PaCO_2$. Nevertheless, this group of patients remains at risk of end-organ damage, cardiac arrest or death if their PaO_2 is allowed to fall too low and their oxygen therapy should be titrated to an initial SpO_2 of 88–92%.

If possible, obtain an arterial blood gas sample for urgent analysis provided this does not delay moving onto assessment of the circulation. This will provide information on the following.

- *Oxygenation, PaO_2*: as a 'rule of thumb', a numerical difference between the PaO_2 (kPa) and inspired oxygen concentration (%) of more than 10 implies a defect in oxygen uptake.
- *Ventilation, $PaCO_2$*: hypercapnia (increased $PaCO_2$) is the result of inadequate alveolar ventilation; hypocapnia, excessive ventilation.
- *Metabolism, pH, base excess*: acutely ill patients usually have a metabolic acidosis (decreased pH, negative base excess or base deficit) in proportion to the severity of illness. An acidosis may also be seen in diabetic ketoacidosis, or in surgical patients who lose bicarbonate via the gastrointestinal tract (for example, diarrhoea, fistulas).
- Many modern blood gas analysers will also measure electrolytes and lactate. An increase in the latter implies significant impairment of tissue oxygenation, even though the PaO_2 may be normal. This signifies a problem with oxygen delivery to the tissues and acute circulatory shock.

Any life-threatening respiratory problem should be treated as soon as it is identified. If the patient's breathing is dangerously inadequate or if the patient is apnoeic, ventilation must be assisted or controlled using a bag-valve-mask with reservoir attached to high-flow oxygen, 15 L/minute, whilst calling urgently for expert help. The addition of a reservoir allows oxygen concentrations close to 100% to be given. For treatment of specific conditions, see later.

 KEY POINTS

- A pulse oximeter does not measure $PaCO_2$ and, therefore, gives no indication of the adequacy of a patient's ventilation.
- Hypoxaemic patients tend to hyperventilate, with a resultant low $PaCO_2$.
- If a patient is receiving oxygen therapy, the SpO_2 may be normal, despite inadequate ventilation.
- A 'normal' PaO_2 (12–14 kPa) whilst breathing 100% oxygen ($FiO_2 \sim 1.0$) is not normal.

Assess the circulation (C)

The aim is to assess the patient's haemodynamic status and to recognize and treat circulatory shock, whatever the cause. Shock is inadequate perfusion of the vital organs with oxygenated blood and if left untreated will lead to ischaemic damage to the vital organs and organ failure. In many surgical and medical emergencies, the cause of shock is hypovolaemia. Major haemorrhage (overt or hidden) should be assumed until proven otherwise in patients who develop shock in the early postoperative period. Respiratory pathology, such as a tension pneumothorax, can also compromise a patient's circulatory state, but should have been detected already and treated if the above system has been followed. The look-listen-feel approach is used again.

Look for:

- the colour of the hands and digits; are they cyanosed, pale or mottled, indicating poor peripheral perfusion?
- fullness of the peripheral veins. Are they underfilled or collapsed, signifying hypovolaemia?
- the central veins. Are they collapsed, signifying hypovolaemia, or engorged, signifying acute left ventricular failure, cardiac tamponade, tension pneumothorax or acute severe asthma?

- other signs of inadequate cardiac output, such as reduced level of consciousness, oliguria (urine volume <0.5 mL/kg/hour);
- obvious signs of blood or extracellular fluid (ECF) loss; bleeding, nasogastric or other drain loss.

NOTE: Empty drains do not exclude active bleeding. Haemorrhage may be concealed (for example, intrathoracic, intraperitoneal, pelvic or into the gut).

Listen for:

- added heart sounds. Third and fourth heart sounds are heard in diastole and result in a triple rhythm – a gallop rhythm. A third heart sound (early diastole) is indicative of heart failure; a fourth heart sound (late diastole) is also indicative of a stiff, poorly functioning left ventricle;
- a heart murmur, usually indicative of valvular heart disease;
- a pericardial rub, indicative of pericarditis;
- very quiet heart sounds, which may be heard in severe emphysema and pericardial effusion.

Feel for:

- limb temperature by feeling the patient's hands and feet. Are they warm or cool, suggesting poor perfusion?
- a central pulse (usually the carotid artery) and compare with a peripheral pulse (usually the radial artery). Assess for:
  - rate;
  - rhythm/regularity;
  - volume;
  - character.

A rapid, weak, low-volume pulse suggests a poor cardiac output. A bounding pulse may indicate sepsis. Measure the patient's blood pressure. The causes of hypotension are listed in Table 9.6.

Finally, measure the capillary refill time (CRT) both centrally and peripherally. Apply firm pressure to a finger-tip or toe for 5 seconds (at heart level or just above) and release: the capillaries should refill (colour returns to the compressed area) in <2 seconds. Capillary refill time may be affected by the environmental temperature. Repeat the procedure over the sternum.

Heart rate and blood pressure must be placed in context; an elderly patient with poor myocardial reserve may be in extremis with a heart rate of 60/minute and blood pressure of 95/60 mmHg, but the same values will be well tolerated or may even be normal for a fit young adult. Ultimately, definitive

Table 9.6 Causes of systemic hypotension.

- Absolute hypovolaemia
  - Dehydration; inadequate input, excessive output
  - Haemorrhage
  - Burns
- Relative hypovolaemia
  - Sepsis
  - Anaphylaxis
  - Spinal cord injury
  - Epidural/spinal anaesthesia
- Cardiogenic
  - Acute myocardial infarction
  - Arrhythmia
  - Severe valvular heart disease
  - Cardiac tamponade
- Obstructive
  - Massive pulmonary embolus
  - Tension pneumothorax
- Drug overdose, e.g. antihypertensives

Table 9.7 Common causes of a decreased conscious level.

- Hypoxaemia
- Hypotension
- Hypercapnia
- Hypoglycaemia
- Hyponatraemia
- Drugs (e.g. sedatives, opiates, overdoses)
- Seizures
- Head injury
- Intracranial haemorrhage
- Cerebral infarction
- Intracranial infection
- Cerebral neoplasm
- Hypothermia
- Hyperthermia
- Hypothyroidism
- Hepatic encephalopathy

treatment of shock will be determined by the cause, the most common being hypovolaemia, sepsis and cardiac failure. These are covered below.

 KEY POINTS

- Resting heart rate is normally lower than systolic blood pressure.
- In some patients, for example those with gastrointestinal or intra-abdominal haemorrhage, immediate surgery may be required as the only effective form of resuscitation.
- Patients with cardiac failure do just as badly if the heart is underfilled as if it is overfilled and so may benefit from intravenous fluids.

Assessing neurological state – disability (D)

The aim is to assess the patient's conscious level, identify any impairment and treat the cause if possible. Common causes of unconsciousness are shown in Table 9.7. Hypoxaemia, hypercapnia or cerebral hypoperfusion should have been detected and treated at an earlier stage of the ABCDE assessment.

Examine the pupils for size and reactivity to light

- Pinpoint pupils, reactive: opioids, pontine lesion.
- Mid-sized, fixed: lesion in the midbrain.
- Dilated, fixed: severe global ischaemia or hypoxia (for example, post cardiac arrest), hypoglycaemia, brainstem lesion, post seizure, drug effects (for example, atropine, adrenaline, overdose of tricyclic antidepressant).
- Unilateral dilatation, fixed: expanding intracranial haematoma causing uncal herniation, lesion of third (oculomotor) cranial nerve.

Other important checks

- Assess the patient's conscious level using the Glasgow Coma Scale (GCS) (Table 9.8) and record the best response.
- Immediately check the patient's glucose using a rapid bedside point of care testing (POCT) blood analyser to exclude severe hypoglycaemia and send blood urgently for more accurate laboratory estimation.
- Check the patient's drug chart for reversible drug-induced causes of depressed consciousness.
- Consider the possibility of acute CNS infection, intracranial haemorrhage or cerebral infarct.
- Status epilepticus should be obvious and treated as described later.

Table 9.8 Glasgow Coma Scale.

Assessment and response	Score
Eye opening	
• Spontaneous	4
• To speech	3
• To pain	2
• None	1
Verbal response	
• Orientated	5
• Confused	4
• Inappropriate words	3
• Incomprehensible sounds	2
• None	1
Best motor response	
• Obeys commands	6
• Localizes to pain	5
• Withdraws from pain	4
• Abnormal flexion to pain	3
• Extension to pain	2
• None	1

Highest achievable score is 15; the lowest score is 3. Coma is defined as a score of 8 or less: patients have no eye opening (1), no verbalization (2), do not obey commands (5).

 KEY POINTS

- Patients who are in coma (GCS <9) are at risk of airway obstruction when supine and airway reflexes may be insufficient to prevent aspiration of secretions, vomit or blood. Nurse in the recovery position and summon expert help to secure their airway.

- If there is a risk of coexisting cervical spine pathology, for example a fracture, nurse the patient supine, maintaining a patent airway. This mandates the constant presence of a nurse or doctor.

- 'Don't Ever Forget Glucose' (DEFG) in any patient with acute deterioration in their conscious level.

Exposure/examination (E)

The aim is to perform a full, head-to-toe, back and front examination of the patient. To allow this, full exposure of the body is necessary, carried out in a way that respects the dignity of the patient and prevents heat loss. Initially, the examination should be focused on the area of the body most likely to be causing the patient's condition; for example, for a patient presenting with shock following a laparotomy, this would be the abdomen. If this step is omitted, vital information regarding the aetiology of the patient's condition may be missed, such as the presence of a purpuric rash signifying meningococcal septicaemia or a knife stab wound in the back of the chest.

What to do next?

The aim so far has been to assess the patient, treat immediately life-threatening problems and produce some clinical improvement, to enable a diagnosis to be made and definitive treatment initiated. Even if the patient's vital signs are still outside the normal range, they should be improving. If not, it is essential to summon senior help and, while waiting for this to arrive, reassess the patient using the ABCDE approach to try and identify the cause.

Once things are improving, gather more information about the patient.

- Take a full history from the patient, staff, relatives or the hospital notes. Comorbid conditions (such as ischaemic heart disease, COPD) can have a significant impact upon a patient's response to critical illness and must not be overlooked.
- If not already done, perform a full examination of the patient, using a traditional clinical examination format.
- Review the patient's notes and charts. Assimilate the data on charts by systematic analysis. Study both absolute values of vital signs and their trends.
- Check that important routine medications are prescribed and being administered. Look for potential interactions.
- Review the results of all laboratory and radiological investigations.

Consider if you have a credible diagnosis that accounts for the patient's condition and recent deterioration:

- if yes, consider the definitive treatment of the patient's underlying condition;
- if no, reassess the patient in case you have missed something important. Involve senior colleagues.

Consider the level of care required by the patient (for example, ward, HDU, ITU); this may be dictated by your hospital's policies. Make complete entries of your findings, assessment and treatment in the patient's notes. Record the patient's response to therapy. Ensure that your entry in the notes is legible, signed, dated and timed.

Communicating information about patient deterioration

Although the systems outlined above will allow the recognition, initial assessment and treatment of the acutely ill patient, on the majority of occasions more senior help will be required to manage the problem safely and effectively. The key to achieving this is good communication at all levels; use either the SBAR or RSVP format (see earlier). Be assertive when communicating, avoid aggression and be honest. 'I am unsure of what to do next' or 'I am worried that I am missing something' are likely to assist in obtaining help.

KEY POINTS

- Always fully expose the patient after ABCD.
- Use a system for communicating patient deterioration, e.g. SBAR or RSVP.

Section 2: Management of common emergencies

Once an initial ABCDE assessment with treatment of immediately life-threatening problems has been performed, attention will need to be focused on determining the underlying problem and beginning appropriate definitive treatment. The following is intended to provide a practical approach to the important aspects of the management of some common emergencies. In most acutely ill patients, initial treatment and investigations will occur simultaneously; they have been separated below for clarity. Clearly, there will frequently be areas of overlap of symptoms and signs; for example, pulmonary embolism may present with shortness of breath, chest pain, hypotension, loss of consciousness or cardiac arrest. In all acute situations get senior help early.

Acute shortness of breath

You will often be called to assess patients who are breathless (dyspnoeic). Respiratory rate is one of the key parameters in all EWS systems and is perhaps the single most sensitive indicator of a potentially life-threatening critical illness. Taking a history from the patient can be challenging if they are too breathless to speak in sentences. This is itself an indicator of an *immediately* life-threatening condition.

There are many causes of acute dyspnoea (see Table 9.5). However, the differential diagnosis can be narrowed by taking into account the history, examination findings and the results of blood tests and other investigations such as chest X-ray and 12-lead ECG. Some of the more common causes of shortness of breath are covered in the following discussion.

Acute upper airway obstruction

If any patient has signs of airway obstruction, **expert help should be called for immediately** (an anaesthetist and, depending on the situation, an ENT surgeon). Common causes are shown in Table 9.3. However, while waiting for help to arrive it is possible to quickly and safely start the process of restoring a patent airway and delivering oxygen. Examine the patient for signs of upper airway obstruction.

Look for:

- distress in the patient;
- use of accessory muscles, often sat upright, flaring of the alae nasi;
- dyspnoea, rapid shallow breaths;
- see-saw or paradoxical respiratory pattern;
- drooling, not swallowing saliva;
- cyanosis.

Listen for:

- abnormal sounds, stridor, wheeze, gurgling;
- reduced or absent breath sounds;
- inability to vocalize, poor voice strength.

Feel for:

- reduced air movement;
- decreased chest expansion;
- pulse rate – this is increased due to hypoxia and hypercapnia.

Other features may be apparent with obstruction due to specific causes and are covered below:

- a reduced conscious level (reduced GCS);
- swelling of the upper airway or tumour;
- external compression of the airway, for example after surgery;
- a blocked tracheostomy or laryngectomy stoma.

Reduced conscious level (reduced GCS score)

This may be either the result of, or the cause of, airway obstruction. In either case, relief of the obstruction is the first step in management.

1 Carry out a visual inspection of the airway and suction any oral/oropharyngeal debris.
2 Open the airway using simple manoeuvres such as head tilt, chin lift and jaw thrust and check for any spontaneous breathing.
3 If breathing is inadequate or absent, use a self-inflating bag with reservoir and face mask attached to 15 L/minute oxygen to assist ventilation.
4 Ventilate by achieving a good seal around the patient's nose and mouth with the facemask and gentle squeezing of the self-inflating bag. This may require a two-person technique.
5 If these basic manoeuvres are inadequate, use a simple airway adjunct, for example using naso- or oropharyngeal airways. If you are trained and it is available, use a supraglottic airway device.
6 Establish basic monitoring including a pulse oximeter, non-invasive blood pressure and three-lead ECG.
7 Once a patent airway and oxygenation is established, check for cardiac output. If it is absent, follow the advanced lifesupport algorithm for cardiac arrest (see later).
8 A suitably trained member of staff may decide that tracheal intubation is needed.

Once the patient has been stabilized with an adequate airway and ventilation and is haemodynamically stable, the next step is to identify the reason for the reduced GCS (see later).

Upper airway swelling/tumour

Swelling of the upper airway may result from infection, allergic reactions, smoke inhalation or ingestion of a caustic liquid. Tumours of the pharynx and larynx may also lead to upper airway obstruction. The cause can often be elicited from an accurate history from the patient, if they are still able to talk, from an accompanying person or the patient's medical notes. Specific findings may include:

- inability to visualize the posterior wall of the oropharynx due to swelling;
- soot in the nares and mouth along with singed facial hair in burns.

Never force a patient with signs of airway obstruction to lie down – gravity may be helping maintain the airway.

The following treatment should be started.

- Give high-flow oxygen via facemask with reservoir.
- Establish basic monitoring including a pulse oximeter, non-invasive blood pressure and three-lead ECG.
- If an inflammatory cause is suspected:
  ○ start treatment with nebulized adrenaline (5 mL 1:1000) in oxygen;
  ○ establish IV access and give 8 mg dexamethasone IV.
- When there is a 'threatened airway':
  ○ nasendoscopy by an experienced operator may provide information about the cause and highlight any potential difficulties with intubation;
  ○ if safe, transfer the patient to either a critical care area or operating theatre;
  ○ an experienced doctor may use 'Heliox', a mixture of oxygen and helium (this reduces the work of breathing), but this will reduce the inspired oxygen concentration.
- If the airway obstructs completely, depending on the skills available:
  ○ attempt oxygenation via facemask and self-inflating bag;
  ○ insert a supraglottic airway, attempt ventilation;
  ○ direct laryngoscopy, attempt tracheal intubation with small-diameter (6 mm) tube;
  ○ perform a surgical airway.
- Once oxygenation is established, transfer to the operating theatre for a definitive airway procedure.

External compression after surgery

There are a number of operations that involve surgical access to, and dissection in, the anterior triangle of the neck – for example thyroidectomy, parathyroidectomy, carotid endarterectomy and cervical disc surgery. The commonest cause of obstruction is development of a haematoma, causing compression of the larynx, displacement of the trachea and laryngeal mucosal engorgement and oedema, all of which lead to airway compromise. Specific findings may include:

- neck swelling;
- bleeding from the wound;
- blocked surgical drain.

More rarely, surgery may inadvertently damage both recurrent laryngeal nerves, causing both cords to adduct and obstruct the airway.

The following treatment should be started.

- Give high-flow oxygen and establish basic monitoring.
- Inform the surgical team; the patient will probably need to be returned to theatre.
- Consider nebulized adrenaline and steroids as described above to reduce any oedema.
- If the neck is obviously swollen, open the surgical incision to allow evacuation of the haematoma and release of the pressure upon the airway.
- Attempt to support ventilation using a facemask and self-inflating bag with 100% oxygen.
- If evacuation of the haematoma does not relieve the obstruction (because of severe laryngeal oedema):
  - direct laryngoscopy by an experienced anaesthetist may allow tracheal intubation;
  - equipment for a surgical airway must be immediately available.

In the case of recurrent laryngeal nerve injury, bag-valve-mask ventilation should be performed initially. Tracheal intubation is usually achievable once hypnotics and a neuromuscular-blocking drug have been given.

Blocked tracheostomy

Tracheostomies are performed for a variety of clinical indications, including upper airway obstruction, to facilitate weaning from mechanical ventilation, to allow long-term ventilation and to provide a route to allow removal of secretions from the patient's respiratory tract. A tracheostomy can be temporary or permanent.

The patient's airway can be compromised because the tube has become either blocked or displaced. Rapid relief of the occlusion usually allows oxygenation but if the tube is displaced it may be the cause of airway obstruction. It may then be necessary to remove the tube to allow the patient to breathe via the tracheostomy track, the normal airway or a combination of both. The management of these patients should follow the published guidelines [9.5] and a summary is shown in Figure 9.3.

In contrast, a laryngectomy is usually performed for carcinoma of the larynx and results in permanent alteration of the patient's airway. These patients are often referred to as 'neck breathers' and rely on their tracheostomy for ventilation. Complications can occur at the time of the procedure (bleeding),

after the procedure (obstruction, displacement) or long term (tracheomalacia, tracheal stenosis). Many of these patients may not have a tracheostomy tube in situ but may have a device to allow 'oesophageal speech'. The management of these patients should follow the published guidelines [9.5] and a summary is shown in Figure 9.4.

Acute lower airway problems

Having assessed and eliminated an upper airway problem as the cause of shortness of breath (see earlier), consideration can be given to lower airway problems. These can be due to primary lung dysfunction or are secondary to other conditions (see Table 9.5). Examine the patient for signs and symptoms of lower airway obstruction.

Look for:

- dyspnoea;
- increased respiratory rate;
- reduced chest expansion;
- use of accessory muscles;
- abdominal breathing pattern;
- tracheal tug.

Listen for:

- rattling or gurgling noises;
- wheeze;
- abnormal breath sounds on auscultation;
- murmurs, additional heart sounds.

Feel for:

- air movement;
- altered percussion note;
- position of the trachea;
- subcutaneous emphysema.

Other features may be apparent with acute lower airway problems due to specific causes and the following are covered in more detail below:

- acute severe asthma;
- pneumonia;
- pneumothorax;
- pulmonary oedema;
- pulmonary embolus.

Acute severe asthma

Although many of the above features may be present, asthma is typically associated with wheeziness. However, when severe, the patient may not be wheezy because of minimal air movement into the chest – the so-called 'silent chest'. Such patients may also be

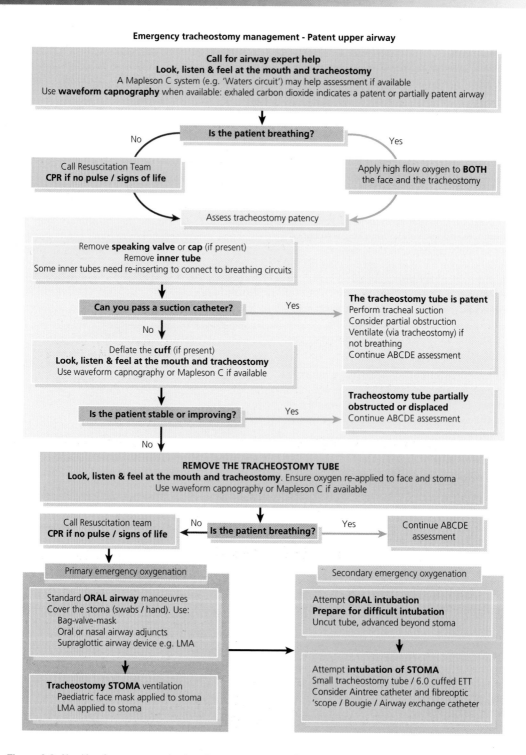

Figure 9.3 Algorithm for emergency tracheostomy management. Source: courtesy of the National Tracheostomy Safety Project.

Emergency laryngectomy management

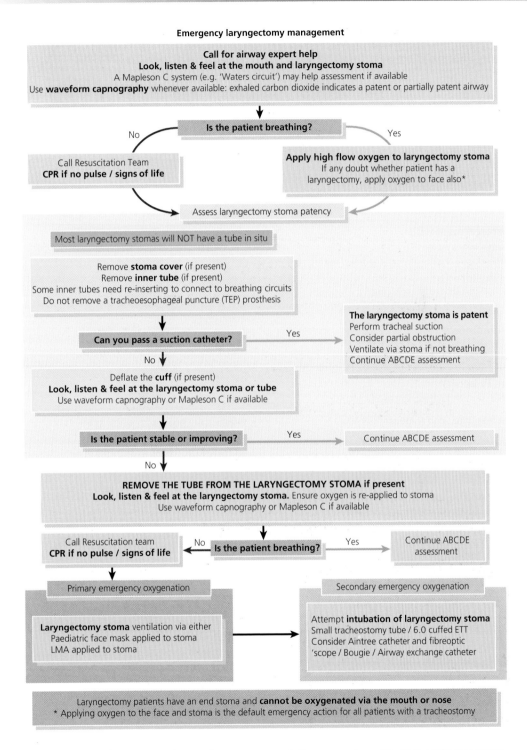

Figure 9.4 Algorithm for emergency laryngectomy management. Source: courtesy of the National Tracheostomy Safety Project.

cyanosed and have a reduced level of consciousness. If any one of the following is present, the patient has acute severe asthma:

- severe breathlessness – unable to complete sentences in one breath;
- respiratory rate >25/minute, heart rate >110/minute;
- if measurable, peak expiratory flow (PEF) 33–50% best or predicted.

The British Thoracic Society (BTS) and Scottish Intercollegiate Guidelines Network (SIGN) have produced guidelines on the management of asthma [9.6].

Start treatment with:
- high-flow oxygen;
- high-dose nebulized beta-2 agonist, salbutamol 5 mg repeated;
- nebulized ipratropium 0.5 mg.

Establish basic monitoring:
- pulse oximetry;
- non-invasive blood pressure;
- three-lead ECG.

Gain IV access:
- give steroids IV, hydrocortisone 100 mg.

If there is little or no response:

- give magnesium sulphate 8 mmol (2 g) slowly IV;
- take an arterial blood sample for blood gas analysis.

Refer to ITU if:
- decreasing peak expiratory flow rate (PEFR) despite treatment;
- increasing hypoxia, $PaO_2 < 8$ kPa;
- hypercapnia, $PaCO_2 > 6.0$ kPa;
- increasing acidosis;
- exhaustion with reduced respiratory effort;
- reduced level of consciousness.

Pneumonia

Pneumonia may be the underlying reason for a patient presenting to hospital, or it may develop during a patient's stay in hospital – for example, atelectasis and sputum retention after abdominal surgery. Pneumonia may develop at any time secondary to aspiration of gastric contents, for example at induction or emergence from anaesthesia, vomiting at any time during impaired consciousness, or due to neuromuscular disorders affecting laryngeal reflexes. On this basis, pneumonia is broadly classified as community-acquired pneumonia (CAP), hospital-acquired pneumonia

(HAP) or aspiration pneumonia. A patient has to have been in hospital for >48 hours prior to the onset of symptoms in order to diagnose HAP. The type of pneumonia has implications for the likely causative pathogens and hence appropriate antimicrobial treatment.

There are three aspects to making the diagnosis of pneumonia.

1 History
Ask specifically about:

- dyspnoea;
- cough;
- pleuritic chest pain;
- purulent sputum;
- high temperature, sweating;
- malaise.

2 Examination
Look for:

- confusion;
- pyrexia;
- dyspnoea at rest, tachypnoea;
- cyanosis, low SpO_2;
- hypotension.

Listen for:

- reduced air entry and possible crackles or bronchial breathing over the affected area, increased vocal resonance and a pleural rub.

Feel for:

- a tachycardia;
- unequal chest expansion;
- percussion – dullness over the affected area (especially if there is an associated effusion).

3 Investigations
- Take blood for full blood count (FBC), urea and electrolytes (U&Es), liver function tests (LFTs), C-reactive protein (CRP) and blood cultures.
- Take an arterial blood sample for blood gas analysis and blood lactate levels. There is often hypoxia with a normal $PaCO_2$, and a metabolic acidosis if the patient is septic.
- Obtain a chest X-ray (CXR). There may be consolidation with loss of volume of one hemithorax, and an associated pleural effusion.

Start treatment
- Oxygen via a facemask, aiming for SpO_2 94–98% (88–92% is acceptable in patients with severe COPD). If there is a large volume of consolidation the SpO_2 may not improve significantly.

Obtain IV access

- Before connecting the IV fluid, take blood for the investigations (see earlier).
- Start IV fluids (Hartmann's solution); give a fluid challenge if hypotensive.
- Commence IV antibiotic therapy according to local policy and likely type of pneumonia – discussion with a microbiologist may be needed.

Start physiotherapy to encourage coughing; consider analgesia for pleuritic chest pain to improve the ability to cough but use caution with the dose of opioids if given.

Establish basic monitoring and record vital signs:

- pulse oximetry, ECG;
- blood pressure (BP), pulse rate;
- respiratory rate;
- temperature;
- GCS score.

Patients with severe pneumonia, or those with pre-existing lung disease, may not respond to initial treatment. Early consideration should be given to ITU admission when the patient shows signs of:

- hypoxaemia, despite a high FiO_2, for example $SpO_2 < 90\%$ or $PaO_2 < 8\,kPa$;
- tiring, becoming drowsy, $PaCO_2$ rising;
- hypotension, not responding to fluid challenges, or a metabolic acidosis (both imply septic shock).

Pneumothorax

This may occur spontaneously (usually in young males) or due to underlying COPD, asthma, lung carcinoma or penetrating chest trauma. A small pneumothorax may be asymptomatic. Specific findings may include complaints of sudden-onset, unilateral, pleuritic chest pain.

Look for:

- dyspnoea;
- unequal chest expansion;
- wounds.

Listen for:

- decreased air entry on the affected side.

Feel for:

- decreased chest expansion on the affected side;
- percussion – hyperresonance on the affected side;
- surgical emphysema.

Start treatment

- High-flow oxygen via facemask with reservoir – this will help limit or reduce the size of the pneumothorax.

Establish basic monitoring:

- pulse oximeter, ECG;
- blood pressure, pulse rate;
- respiratory rate;
- GCS score.

Gain IV access:

- start slow infusion of fluid;
- give analgesia if required.

Investigations

- Arrange CXR:
  - if pneumothorax is >20% radiographic lung volume, aspirate air;
  - under strict asepsis and local anaesthesia, insert a 16 G needle into the chest in the second intercostal space, midclavicular line;
  - connect to a 50 mL syringe via a three-way tap;
  - aspirate up to 2.5 L air or until the patient starts to cough or resistance is felt.
- Repeat CXR after attempt to drain the pneumothorax.

If the pneumothorax recurs, it will need drainage via a tube thoracostomy.

Tension pneumothorax

Occasionally, the volume of air in the pleural cavity increases rapidly, because it is sucked in during inspiration, because it fails to escape during expiration, or air is forced in during positive pressure ventilation. It is most commonly associated with trauma but may occur after insertion of a central venous pressure (CVP) line if the needle accidentally punctures the pleura. The effect is a gradual increase in intrathoracic pressure, initially causing the lung to collapse followed by shift of the mediastinum, impaired venous return and cardiovascular collapse. This is an immediately life-threatening condition and unless treated urgently will cause cardiac arrest. Specific findings include:

- severe respiratory distress, markedly tachypnoeic;
- distended neck veins (only if the patient is not hypovolaemic);
- decreased movement of one hemithorax – it may appear hyperinflated and immobile;
- absent breath sounds on the affected side;
- hyperresonance on the affected side;
- tachycardia and hypotension;
- tracheal deviation away from the affected side – usually a pre-arrest finding;
- cyanosis.

Start treatment
- Give high-flow oxygen via facemask with reservoir.
- Gain IV access, start a rapid fluid bolus.
- If the patient is in extremis, if the skills/equipment to perform a thoracostomy are not immediately available, insert a 14 G or 16 G needle into the chest in the second intercostal space, midclavicular line on the affected side. This is a temporizing measure only.
- As soon as safe, perform a thoracostomy in the fifth intercostal space, midaxillary line, on the affected side and arrange for insertion of a tube thoracostomy.
- Arrange for CXR.

 KEY POINT

- Do not delay decompression of the chest by requesting an X-ray. Tension pneumothorax is a clinical diagnosis.

Pulmonary oedema

Although a small amount of fluid normally passes from pulmonary capillaries into the interstitial space of the lungs, the alveoli of the lungs are normally 'dry' and this interstitial fluid is drained off via the lymphatic system. However, when the rate of transcapillary fluid migration is excessive, the lymphatic system cannot accommodate it and both interstitial and alveolar oedema develops. Although the list of possible causes of pulmonary oedema is long (Table 9.9), pulmonary oedema is commonly associated with two conditions:

- an increase in the transcapillary hydrostatic pressure seen in left ventricular failure (LVF);
- an increase in pulmonary capillary permeability seen in severe sepsis and acute respiratory distress syndrome (ARDS).

The following is based on treating a patient with pulmonary oedema secondary to acute LVF. When examining a patient, pulmonary oedema is suggested by a number of clinical findings.

Look for:
- signs of respiratory failure:
  - dyspnoea;
  - tachypnoea;
  - central cyanosis or pallor;
- cough with pink, frothy sputum;
- sweating;
- distended neck veins (raised jugular venous pressure).

Table 9.9 Causes of pulmonary oedema.

Increased transcapillary pressure	Increased capillary permeability
• ACS	• Severe sepsis
• Severe bradycardia	• Aspiration pneumonitis
• Severe tachycardia	• Acute pancreatitis
• Severe valvular heart disease	• Major trauma
• Fluid overload, e.g. iatrogenic, renal failure	• Massive blood transfusion
• Infective endocarditis/ myocarditis	• ABO blood group incompatible transfusion
• Pericardial effusion/ cardiac tamponade	• Embolism: fat or amniotic fluid
	• Burns: cutaneous or inhalational injury

ACS, acute coronary syndrome.

Listen for:
- fine, inspiratory crackles/crepitations;
- wheeze;
- the presence of additional heart sounds (gallop rhythm);
- heart murmurs.

Feel for:
- displaced apex beat;
- apical heave.

Start treatment
- Give high-flow oxygen therapy using a facemask and attached reservoir bag at a flow rate of 15 L/minute.
- Sit the patient as upright as possible; this reduces venous return to the heart, pulmonary capillary pressure and left ventricular filling pressure.

Establish basic monitoring:
- pulse oximeter, ECG;
- blood pressure, pulse rate;
- respiratory rate;
- GCS score.

Gain IV access
- Give intravenous diuretics (for example, furosemide 20–100 mg in divided doses); this causes vasodilatation and reduces preload and

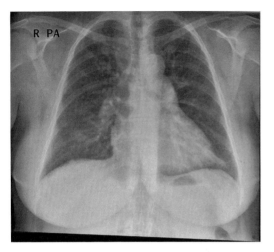

R PA

Figure 9.5 Chest X-ray showing acute pulmonary oedema.

afterload, followed by a diuresis, which again reduces preload.

- Additional preload reduction can be produced by an intravenous infusion of nitrates, such as isosorbide dinitrate. The infusion is usually started at 2 mg/hour and gradually increased in increments to the maximum rate possible whilst still maintaining systolic blood pressure >100 mmHg.
- Carefully titrated IV diamorphine (up to 5 mg in 1 mg aliquots); this reduces anxiety and excessive sympathetic nervous system activity and also provides further vasodilatation.

Investigations
- CXR: may be pathognomonic of pulmonary oedema and is key to a firm diagnosis (Figure 9.5).
- Twelve-lead ECG: this is essential to confirm or refute the possibility of an acute coronary syndrome (ACS) as the cause (see Figure 9.7).

Further measures
- Continuous positive airway pressure (CPAP) via a facemask may be beneficial and is sometimes available on acute medical wards. It improves oxygenation by:
  - increasing the functional residual capacity (FRC), reducing the work of breathing;
  - reopening closed and underventilated alveoli (recruitment), thereby reducing intrapulmonary shunting;
  - reducing left ventricular preload and afterload, reducing the degree of heart failure.

- If the patient does not improve with these measures, consideration should be given to treating with an inotrope (for example, dobutamine), particularly if hypotension is also present.
- Carefully selected patients may be transferred to the critical care unit for invasive ventilation.

Pulmonary embolism

This is a common cause of morbidity and mortality in hospitalized patients, the majority of which can be prevented through adequate risk stratification and prophylaxis as described in Chapter 1. Despite these measures, some patients will still go on to develop a pulmonary embolism (PE), which can present with collapse and pulseless electrical activity (PEA) cardiac arrest. The probability of the patient having had a PE can be assessed using the Wells score. A numeric value is assigned to the following criteria; the greater the sum, the greater probability of a PE:

- surgery or immobilization within the previous four weeks;
- malignancy;
- previous history of deep venous thrombosis (DVT)/pulmonary embolism;
- haemoptysis;
- tachycardia, >100/minute;
- clinical symptoms of a DVT;
- alternative diagnosis less likely than PE.

On assessment, identify specific features suggesting a PE.

Look for:
- signs of respiratory failure;
- distended neck veins;
- clinical evidence of a DVT.

Listen for:
- pleural rub;
- heart murmur associated with acute tricuspid regurgitation;
- additional heart sounds (gallop rhythm), widely split second heart sound.

Feel for:
- tachycardia and hypotension;
- pulsus paradoxus.

Other findings include:
- chest pain;
- haemoptysis;
- pyrexia;
- syncope;
- (specific ECG changes – see later).

Start treatment

This will depend, to an extent, on the severity of the PE.

- All patients should initially be given oxygen therapy using a facemask and attached reservoir bag at a flow rate of 15 L/minute.
- Many patients will require analgesia.
- All patients will require anticoagulation with either subcutaneous low molecular weight heparin or an intravenous infusion of unfractionated heparin until the diagnosis is confirmed/excluded and oral anticoagulation therapy established if appropriate.

In severe cases

- Secure venous access (16 G cannula or larger); give a fluid challenge, 500 mL of warmed crystalloid or colloid. This should be repeated up to a volume of 2 L if a satisfactory response is not obtained.
- Inotropes or vasopressors may be necessary in a periarrest situation to support the circulation. This will require urgent advice from critical care specialists.
- Intravenous thrombolytic therapy should be initiated if there are signs of circulatory collapse, such as severe hypotension or arrhythmia, and only after exclusion of other diagnoses which would render such treatment dangerous.

The BTS has published guidelines on the management of suspected acute pulmonary embolism (see Further information).

Investigations

- *Chest X-ray*: often unremarkable although occasionally one or both pulmonary arteries appear prominent and a peripheral wedge-shaped abnormality in one of the lung fields may be secondary to pulmonary infarction. There may be loss of the costophrenic angle due to a small effusion.
- *ECG*: the commonest abnormality is sinus tachycardia. Specific features suggesting right heart strain and the classic S1, Q3, T3 pattern are rarely seen, and have a low negative predictive value when absent.
- *Arterial blood gas analysis* will show hypoxaemia and hypocapnia in cases of significant pulmonary embolism but this is relatively non-specific.
- *D-dimer (a fibrin degradation product) assay*: almost always raised in cases of acute pulmonary embolism. Unfortunately, there are other causes for increased D-dimer. A negative result usually rules out the diagnosis.

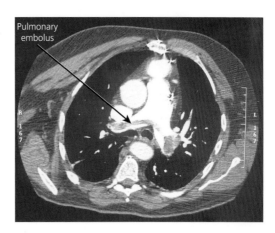

Figure 9.6 CT pulmonary angiogram showing 'saddle' embolus in the pulmonary artery.

- *Imaging*: definitive diagnosis may require ventilation perfusion scan or CT pulmonary angiography (CTPA) (Figure 9.6). Echocardiography, which can be performed at the patient's bedside, will show abnormalities of the right heart in around half of all patients with significant pulmonary embolism.

Hypotension

This is a common reason for being called to see an acutely unwell patient, particularly in the postoperative period. Blood pressure is measured in all patients routinely and is a key element in all EWS systems, but surprisingly, it is not a particularly sensitive or specific indicator of the presence of a life-threatening problem unless the value is extremely high or low.

There are many causes of hypotension (see Table 9.6) but, as with disturbances of other systems, diagnosis of the cause can be determined by taking into account the history, examination findings and results of investigations. After elimination of airway and breathing problems as a cause for the hypotension, examine the patient for the following signs and symptoms.

Look for:

- evidence of impaired cerebral perfusion; conscious level:
  - orientated – good;
  - confused/agitated – bad;
  - unresponsive – worse;
- tachypnoea, dyspnoea;
- colour: pale, cyanosed, flushed;

- sweating;
- neck veins: collapsed or distended (raised jugular venous pressure).

Listen for:

- abnormal breath sounds; fine inspiratory crackles and/or (cardiac) wheeze;
- the presence of additional heart sounds (gallop rhythm) or a murmur;
- altered or absent breath sounds.

Feel for:

- pulse: rate, volume (central – for example carotid, femoral – and peripheral, for example radial, dorsalis pedis) and regularity;
- capillary refill time:
  - firm pressure applied over the sternum (central refill time) and to a digit (peripheral refill time) for 5 seconds to produce blanching;
  - prompt return of colour within 2 seconds maximum is normal;
  - delayed peripheral capillary refill suggests a low cardiac output and/or perfusion pressure, delayed central capillary refill is an ominous sign;
  - unreliable in hypothermic patients;
- position of the apex beat;
- position of the trachea.

Finally, look at the patient's fluid balance chart, in particular the urine output over the previous 12 hours.

These patients are often referred to as being in 'shock'. Strictly speaking, shock is defined as 'inadequate perfusion of the tissues with oxygenated blood' and although hypotension is a common feature, it may not always be present initially. Because of its common usage, the following types of shock are covered in more detail below:

- hypovolaemic shock;
- septic shock;
- anaphylactic shock;
- cardiogenic shock.

Hypovolaemic shock

Common causes of hypovolaemia include bleeding (external or concealed), excessive losses from the gastrointestinal tract (for example, diarrhoea, vomiting, fistula loss), excessive third space losses after major tissue trauma and the relative hypovolaemia that occurs with epidural anaesthesia. The latter two causes are covered in Chapter 8.

Specific findings in hypovolaemia are manifestations of the increase in sympathetic outflow:

- vasoconstriction, causing pallor, peripheral cyanosis, cold extremities, delayed capillary refill;
- empty peripheral veins;
- tachycardia;
- sweating;
- narrowing of the pulse pressure;
- oliguria.

In the postsurgery patient, ongoing haemorrhage will be suggested by:

- a large volume of blood in the surgical drains, or from a wound;
- a distending abdomen;
- wound swelling.

Start treatment

- All patients should be given oxygen via a facemask and reservoir at a flow rate of 15 L/minute.
- In all cases, obtain large-bore venous access (14 or 16 G cannula). The antecubital fossa is often the best site for the largest vein. In severe hypovolaemia, two cannulas should be inserted, one on either side. Before connecting the IV fluid, take blood for the investigations (see later).
- Give a rapid fluid challenge (over 5–10 minutes):
  - 250 mL of warmed crystalloid solution (for example, 0.9% saline or Hartmann's solution) if the patient's systolic blood pressure (SBP) is >100 mmHg;
  - 500 mL of warmed crystalloid solution if the patient's SBP is <100 mmHg;
  - 250 mL of warmed crystalloid solution if the patient has pre-existing cardiac failure.
  The choice of fluid (crystalloid versus colloid) is not as important as the fact that some fluid is being given. Avoid dextrose-containing fluids, as they rapidly distribute throughout the total body water and have minimal intravascular effect. In addition, they cause hyperglycaemia, which is associated with increased mortality in critically ill patients.
- Reassess the pulse rate and blood pressure regularly (every 5 minutes), watching for signs of improvement: decreased pulse rate, increased blood pressure, improved level of consciousness. If not already done, consider inserting a urinary catheter. A urine output of 0.5–1.0 mL/kg/hour suggests adequate vital organ perfusion.
- Repeat the fluid challenge if the response is unsatisfactory.
- Arterial blood gas analysis will be useful in determining the net pathophysiological effect of the patient's shock. Metabolic acidosis signified by low pH, high negative base excess and elevated

serum lactate is found proportionate to the severity and duration of the shock state. Serial assays are useful in assessing response to treatment.

- Call for urgent senior help if the patient is not responding. Even if the patient has a satisfactory response to the fluid challenge, help will often still be required for definitive treatment.
- Increasingly, transthoracic echocardiography (TTE) is being used to diagnose a number of problems including hypovolaemia (reduced ventricular filling) and left ventricular dysfunction (see later).
- Acute haemorrhage, which may be overt or covert, must be controlled and this may require the urgent transfer of the patient to the operating theatre or interventional radiology. The resuscitation fluid in these circumstances is blood; however, haemostasis has a higher priority than restoration of a normal blood pressure. Rapid, high-volume fluid resuscitation will exacerbate bleeding and is associated with a worse prognosis.
- Hypotensive resuscitation requires the judgement of an experienced clinician.

Investigations
- FBC, U&Es, blood glucose, CRP, coagulation screen, blood cultures (if indicated).
- Blood grouping and cross-match in case of need for transfusion.
- Twelve-lead ECG to identify any arrhythmia or ischaemia.
- CXR to identify haemothorax, pneumothorax, heart failure, infection.
- Arterial blood gas analysis to assess oxygenation, ventilation, acid–base status.
- Ultrasound assessment of abdomen and/or chest to identify free fluid.
- Send samples of faeces for microbiological assessment.

In patients with suspected cardiac failure, early consideration should be given to invasive monitoring, for example CVP. Early use of direct arterial pressure measurement is also valuable (Table 9.10). It is now possible to use an arterial line to monitor cardiac output using a technique known as pulse contour analysis (see Chapter 3).

Sepsis and septic shock

The pathophysiology of hypotension due to sepsis is entirely different to hypovolaemic or cardiogenic shock. Any major insult to the body, such as infection,

Table 9.10 Advantages and disadvantages of direct arterial blood pressure measurement.

Advantages
- Accuracy (particularly at extremes of high and low pressure)
- Continuous measurement gives immediate warning of important changes in blood pressure
- Shape of arterial waveform gives information relating to myocardial contractility and other haemodynamic variables
- Facility for frequent arterial blood sampling

Disadvantages
- Requires expertise for insertion and subsequent care
- Potentially inaccurate if apparatus is not set up correctly
- Haematoma at puncture site
- Infection at puncture site/bacteraemia/septicaemia
- Disconnection haemorrhage
- Embolization
- Arterial thrombosis

major trauma, burns or acute pancreatitis, initiates a hypermetabolic, inflammatory state termed the 'systemic inflammatory response syndrome' (SIRS). The diagnosis of SIRS is based on finding two or more of the following:

- temperature >38 °C or <36 °C;
- heart rate >90 beats/minute;
- respiratory rate >20 breaths/minute or $PaCO_2 < 4.2\,kPa$;
- white blood cell (WBC) count >12 000/mm³, <4000/mm³ or >10% immature (band) forms.

Sepsis is a condition in which SIRS is due to documented or suspected infection. When the infection overwhelms the patient's immune system, there is systemic spread via the bloodstream (septicaemia). This triggers an inflammatory cascade, the production of inflammatory mediators that cause intense vasodilatation, capillary leak and maldistribution of blood flow at the microcirculatory level. The reflex response is an increase in sympathetic discharge causing tachycardia, increase in stroke volume and cardiac output. Despite this response, there may still be hypotension (SBP <90 mmHg) and evidence of hypoperfusion (serum lactate >2 mmol/L, oliguria <0.5 mL/kg/hour); this defines severe sepsis. Septic shock is a subset of severe sepsis where there is persistent arterial hypotension (SBP <90 mmHg) and perfusion abnormalities despite adequate fluid resuscitation (serum lactate >4 mmol/L).

Failure to recognize and treat septic shock will result in progression to 'multiple organ dysfunction syndrome' (MODS) – the presence of altered organ function such that normal homeostasis cannot be maintained without intervention such as mechanical ventilation or renal replacement therapy. The signs of septic shock are typically:

- pyrexia;
- tachypnoea;
- warm, flushed peripheries with normal capillary refill time (CRT);
- tachycardia;
- a bounding pulse with a wide pulse pressure;
- oliguria.

Start treatment

This is based on the Surviving Sepsis Campaign bundles [9.7].

To be completed within 3 hours of presentation or diagnosis of severe sepsis.

- Give high-flow oxygen.
- Obtain blood cultures before giving antibiotics.
- Measure lactate.
- Give broad-spectrum antibiotics.
- Give boluses of fluid, 250–500 mL of crystalloid, to a maximum of 30 mL/kg if hypotensive or if serum lactate >2 mmol/L.

To be completed within 6 hours.

- Start vasopressors to maintain mean arterial pressure (MAP) >65 mmHg (if hypotension has not responded to fluid resuscitation).
- If persistently hypotensive after fluid resuscitation or lactate >4 mmol/L, undertake further assessment of volume and tissue perfusion status with:
  - clinical examination;
  - bedside echo;
  - insertion of a central line and measurement of CVP or ScvO$_2$;
  - response to a fluid challenge or passive leg raise.
- Remeasure lactate.

Early antibiotic therapy is strongly associated with improved survival and is even more important than fluid resuscitation. Mortality from serve sepsis increases by approximately 7% for every hour of delay in starting antibiotics.

Loss of fluid through leaky capillaries has traditionally lead to excessively high volumes of acute resuscitation fluids – sometimes over 5 L over a period of several hours. Continual fluid infusion will inevitably lead to pulmonary interstitial and alveolar oedema, respiratory distress and hypoxaemia – acute respiratory distress syndrome (ARDS). There is now increasing awareness of this and a move towards earlier use of vasopressors following initial fluid resuscitation (usually after approximately 2000 mL). Those patients who do not show an improvement in tissue perfusion with fluid resuscitation (those with septic shock) will need to be managed in a critical care unit where vasopressors can be used and invasive haemodynamic monitoring can be instituted.

Anaphylaxis

Most adverse drug reactions in anaesthesia are mild and transient, consisting mainly of localized urticaria as a result of cutaneous histamine release. The incidence of anaphylaxis caused by anaesthetic drugs is between 1:10 000 and 1:20 000 drug dosages, and is more common in females. Of those incidents reported to the Medicines Control Agency, 10% involved a fatality compared to 3.7% for drugs overall. This probably reflects the frequency with which anaesthetic drugs are given intravenously. Clinical features include (in order of frequency):

- severe hypotension;
- severe bronchospasm;
- skin changes – erythema, urticaria;
- angio-oedema, which may involve the airway;
- pruritus, nausea and vomiting;
- hypoxaemia.

 KEY POINT

- Skin changes alone are not a sign of anaphylaxis.

Cardiovascular collapse is the most common and severe feature. Asthmatics often develop bronchospasm that is resistant to treatment and are at a greater risk of death, especially when the asthma is poorly controlled or there is a delay in treatment. Any circumstance that reduces the patient's catecholamine response (such as beta-blockers, spinal anaesthesia) will increase the severity.

Anaphylaxis involves the degranulation of mast cells and basophils, as the result of either an allergic (IgE mediated) or non-allergic (non-IgE mediated) reaction, liberating histamine, 5-hydroxytryptamine (5-HT) and associated vasoactive substances. The latter used to be called an anaphylactoid reaction, but this term is no longer used. The European Academy of Allergology and Clinical Immunology Nomenclature Committee has proposed the following broad definition:

Anaphylaxis is a severe, life-threatening generalized or systemic hypersensitivity reaction.

Causes of allergic reactions

Overall, the commonest triggers are foods, drugs, stinging insects and latex. During anaesthesia the commonest triggers are as follows.

- *Anaesthetic drugs:*
  - muscle relaxants (~60%): suxamethonium, rocuronium, atracurium, vecuronium;
  - induction agents (5%): thiopentone, propofol.
- *Latex* (20%).
- *Antibiotics* (15%):
  - penicillin (70% of all antibiotic-related anaphylaxis);
  - <1% of penicillin-allergic patients may cross-react to modern cephalosporins.
- *Intravenous fluids:* colloids (3%).
- *Opioids* (2%).

Immediate management

The following advice is based on guidelines issued by the Resuscitation Council (UK) [9.8].

- Discontinue all drugs likely to have triggered the reaction.
- Call for help.
- Maintain a patent airway, give high-flow oxygen.
- Elevate the patient's legs providing ventilation is not compromised.
- Give adrenaline, 50 µg *slowly* intravenously (0.5 mL of 1:10 000) under ECG control. Dilution of adrenaline to 1:100 000 (10 µg/mL) allows better titration and reduces the risk of adverse effects. If no ECG available, give 0.5 mg intramuscularly (0.5 mL of 1:1000). If there is no improvement within 5 minutes, give a further dose.
- Ensure adequate ventilation: intubation will be required if spontaneous ventilation is inadequate or in the presence of severe bronchospasm. This may be exceedingly difficult in the presence of severe laryngeal oedema. In these circumstances a needle cricothyroidotomy or surgical airway will be required.
- Support the circulation: start a rapid IV infusion of fluids 10–20 mL/kg. Crystalloids initially may be safer than colloids. In the absence of a major pulse,

start cardiopulmonary resuscitation using the appropriate protocol (see later).
- Monitoring:
  - ECG, SpO_2, blood pressure, end-tidal CO_2. Establish an arterial line and check the blood gases:
  - monitor CVP and urine output to assess adequacy of circulating volume.

Subsequent management

- *Antihistamines:* chlorpheniramine (H1 blocker) 10–20 mg slowly IV or IM. There is no evidence for the use of H2 blockers.
- *Steroids:* hydrocortisone 200 mg slowly IV or IM. This helps to reduce late sequelae.
- *Bronchodilators:* salbutamol, 2.5–5.0 mg nebulized or 0.25 mg IV, ipratroprium 500 µg. Magnesium 2 g (8 mmol) slowly IV may be useful when there are severe, asthma-like features or if the patient is taking beta-blockers. Magnesium may cause flushing and may worsen hypotension.

As soon as possible, these patients should be transferred to an ITU for further treatment and monitoring. Reactions vary in severity, can be biphasic, delayed in onset (particularly latex sensitivity) and prolonged. An infusion of adrenaline may be required. The possibility of a tension pneumothorax (secondary to barotrauma) causing hypotension must not be forgotten.

Investigations

The most informative is measurement of plasma mast cell tryptase levels. A blood sample should be taken immediately after treatment and repeated approximately 1–2 hours and 24 hours after the event. Elevated tryptase levels confirm that the reaction was associated with mast cell degranulation but does not distinguish between an allergic and non-allergic cause. A negative test does not completely exclude anaphylaxis. Expert advice about follow-up and identification of the cause must be arranged.

Finally, record all details in the patient's notes, and do not forget to inform the patient and the patient's general practitioner of the events, both verbally and in writing. In the UK, report adverse drug events to the Medicines and Healthcare products Regulatory Agency by completing a 'yellow card' found in the BNF.

Generalized atopy does not help predict the risk of immunologically mediated reaction to anaesthetic drugs. A previous history of 'allergy to an anaesthetic' is cause for concern and there is a high risk of cross-reactivity between drugs of the same group. These patients must be investigated appropriately [9.9].

Cardiogenic shock

Patients with cardiogenic shock due to acute heart failure associated with an acute coronary syndrome (ACS) are managed differently, so it is essential to make the correct diagnosis. This will often come from the clinical context of the patient's illness and any typical physical signs present. Management of the hypotension and management of the ACS are covered in the relevant sections later in this chapter.

Most patients with cardiogenic shock will present with left ventricular failure that can be described as one of the following.

- 'Forward failure' – a decrease in stroke volume and cardiac output. Symptoms and signs include pallor, peripheral cyanosis, cold extremities, delayed capillary refill, oliguria, altered conscious level and gallop rhythm.
- 'Backward failure' – acute dilatation of the left side of the heart and accumulation of blood in the pulmonary circulation that promotes the development of acute pulmonary oedema. Symptoms and signs include dyspnoea, wheeze, cough with pink frothy sputum, cyanosis, basal crackles in the lungs and displaced apex beat.

Frequently, both types of failure coexist.

- In some patients with acute inferior myocardial infarction when the predominant problem may be failure of the right rather than the left ventricle. Symptoms and signs include peripheral oedema, jugular vein distension, hepatomegaly (tender), ascites and pleural effusion.

Start treatment
- This will consist initially of treatment of pulmonary oedema as described earlier.
- Patients with poor cardiac output are not usually hypovolaemic and do not respond favourably to a fluid challenge as this compounds the problem of excessive filling pressure.
- Inotropic support with dobutamine may be required to improve contractility of the left ventricle and this will necessitate the patient being transferred to a critical or coronary care unit for invasive monitoring.
- Where monitoring can be used to confirm adequate or excessive left ventricular filling pressures, diuretic and vasodilator therapy can be used to improve cardiac output.
- Patients with predominant right heart failure are the exception to the withhold fluids rule – poor performance of the right ventricle leads to underfilling of the left ventricle and a fluid challenge may be beneficial.

Investigations
- CXR may show cardiomegaly, pulmonary congestion, Kerley B lines, loss of costophrenic angles.
- Twelve-lead ECG may show evidence of ischaemia or an arrhythmia (see later).
- Echocardiography will reveal left and right ventricular dysfunction (ischaemia, cardiomyopathy) or valvular disease.
- Blood tests as above plus markers of myocardial infarction (cardiac troponins).

Low urine output

The obligatory minimum daily urine output consistent with maintaining normal homeostasis is approximately 500 mL. If urine output falls below this level, or if the kidneys are incapable of producing urine of appropriate concentration for the volume produced, renal failure results [9.10]. Oliguria is usually defined as <0.5 mL/kg/hour. Anuria is the complete absence of urine production; this cannot be diagnosed with certainty unless the patient is catheterized. However, it is essential to recognize that the commonest cause of anuria in an already catheterized patient is a blocked catheter! Palpation over the lower abdomen of an anuric, catheterized patient may confirm the diagnosis. Regardless, the urinary catheter of all such patients should be either flushed or replaced.

For patients on general wards, the most important causes of oliguria are:

- hypovolaemia, usually as a result of:
  - inadequate fluid intake to meet needs;
  - losses from drains, gastrointestinal tract (vomiting, diarrhoea, fistulas);
  - third space losses after major surgery;
  - haemorrhage;
  - sepsis.
- stress response to surgery (see Chapter 8).

Failure to recognize and treat hypovolaemia will lead to the development of pre-renal acute kidney injury (AKI). If diagnosed and treated promptly, particularly with sufficient volume resuscitation, pre-renal AKI often resolves and urine output increases. The aetiology of AKI can also be renal or postrenal. The causes are summarized in Table 9.11.

Similarly, postrenal AKI is potentially reversible if recognized early enough and the obstruction relieved, which may be as simple as catheterizing the patient.

Table 9.11 Aetiology of acute kidney injury.

Pre-renal
- Dehydration, e.g. vomiting, diarrhoea
- Haemorrhage
- Cardiogenic shock
- 'Third space losses', e.g. trauma, major surgery, bowel obstruction
- Sepsis
- Burns

Renal
- Acute tubular necrosis (usually secondary to severe pre-renal failure)
- Sepsis
- Severe obstructive jaundice
- Blood transfusion reaction
- Myoglobinaemia secondary to ischaemic muscle damage and rhabdomyolysis
- Acute glomerular disorders
- Infection, e.g. acute pyelonephritis
- Vasculitis

Postrenal
- Bilateral obstruction to renal outflow (e.g. tumour)

Table 9.12 Differentiation of pre-renal from intrinsic renal failure.

Index	Pre-renal	Intrinsic renal
Urine concentration	High	Dilute
Specific gravity	≥ 1020	<1010
Osmolarity (mosmol/L)	>550	<350
Urine (Na) (mmol/L)	<20	>40
Urine/plasma osmolar ratio	$\geq 2:1$	$1.1:1$
Urine/plasma (urea)	$\geq 20:1$	$<10:1$
Urine/plasma (creatinine)	$\geq 40:1$	$<10:1$
Plasma (urea) (mmol/L)/ (creatinine) (μmol/L) ratio	>0.1	<0.1

Patients suffering from an inadequate fluid intake will have signs and symptoms of dehydration, the severity of which will depend on the fluid deficit:

- <10% loss body weight:
  - thirst, dry mouth;
  - tachycardia;
  - empty peripheral and central veins (low CVP);
  - reduced skin turgor;
- >10% loss body weight: as above plus increased respiratory rate, hypotension, anuria, delirium, coma.

A review of the patient's fluid balance charts will often reveal trends of increasing pulse rate, decreasing urine output, falling blood pressure and increasing respiratory rate.

Start treatment
When asked to see a patient on the ward who is oliguric, the initial approach must be directed at identifying and treating any airway, breathing and circulation problems.

- *Hypoxaemia:* immediate treatment with oxygen as described earlier.

- *Hypotension:* identify the likely cause and treat as described earlier. In most cases this will require fluid resuscitation. There will be a delay after appropriate resuscitation has been provided before urine production increases – resist the temptation to give a dose of a diuretic, for example furosemide, which does not have a useful place in the treatment of pre-renal failure.
- *Exclude a postrenal cause urgently:* this is usually done by excluding urinary retention clinically, ensuring that a urinary catheter, if present, is not blocked.
- *Stop all nephrotoxic drugs:* these include NSAIDs, aminoglycosides and angiotensin converting enzyme (ACE) inhibitors. Paracetamol is safe in the acute setting.

Any condition that precipitated acute pre-renal failure must be treated, for example sepsis secondary to perforated abdominal viscus requires urgent surgical referral for a laparotomy. Once these have been eliminated or treated, follow current guidelines [9.11].

Investigations
- FBC will usually show an increased haematocrit due to dehydration and raised white cell count if infection is present.
- Plasma U&Es and creatinine: will normally show an increase in plasma sodium and urea but little increase in creatinine.
- Urine sodium is reduced (Table 9.12).
- Plasma and urine osmolalities will show a high urinary to plasma osmolality, often >1.5:1.
- Ultrasound of the kidneys and ureters to exclude obstruction to urine flow.

GA: drug-induced, reversible state - loss of consc, loss of awareness and recall of noxious stimuli.

Balanced GA →

loss of cons.

△

analgesia   muscle relax.

Balance of all so ↓ need of single agent → SE.

Transfer: ↑ vigilance, vital signs, End-tidal CO_2, ECG, pressure points, position. All drug before prepping.

Multimodal analgesia: local infiltration - Sx

Simple analgesia - Paracetamol

Bolus of opioid - morphine, reni

RA

As stated earlier, failure to recognize and treat these problems will lead to AKI and the development of acute tubular necrosis (ATN). Diagnosis is predominantly based on the history and investigations:

- taking a blood sample for U&Es and creatinine;
- estimated glomerular filtration rate (eGFR);
- measured creatinine clearance;
- urinalysis.

Raised serum urea and creatinine are synonymous with renal failure. However, it is important to be wary of several pitfalls.

- Normal values may not be normal for specific patient groups. A frail, elderly patient's serum creatinine concentration may be within normal limits, but may in fact reflect abnormal renal function.
- A single U&E estimation is a snapshot of renal function and is only reliable when renal function is stable. A patient who has become acutely oliguric may have normal values.
- Many laboratories provide an estimate of GFR (eGFR). This is estimated using an algorithm based often only on the patient's age, sex and weight. It is not valid in an acute situation where the serum creatinine is in the process of either rising or falling.
- Renal function has to be severely impaired for the numbers to change. Serum creatinine only starts to rise significantly above the normal range when GFR falls below about 30 mL/minute (normal 125 mL/minute). A modestly elevated creatinine indicates quite severe loss of global renal function.
- There could be other reasons for a rising urea; in dehydrated patients a urea concentration relatively higher than the creatinine may indicate dehydration without AKI. In upper GI bleeding, high levels of protein breakdown lead to increased urea production with raised serum concentrations. All of these conditions also predispose to AKI.

Urinalysis will show dilute urine, with a low osmolality (urine:plasma ratio, 1.1:1) (see Table 9.12). Urine microscopy may show the presence of casts (indicative of ATN and glomerulonephritis) and microorganisms (urinary sepsis is a common cause of AKI). However, urinalysis is not useful for diagnosing whether or not pre-renal failure is the cause (see Table 9.12).

A patient with raised serum urea and creatinine who is developing or has established acute renal failure should be transferred to a critical care unit to allow central venous pressure, direct arterial pressure and cardiac output monitoring. These will guide fluid therapy more reliably. If required, the patient can be commenced on renal replacement therapy (RRT) with continuous veno-venous haemofiltration, an extracorporeal renal support therapy similar in some ways to the more familiar intermittent haemodialysis.

If pre-renal and postrenal causes are excluded, there is likely to be a significant intrinsic renal problem. These patients will require urgent specialist nephrologist help with investigation and management.

Chest pain

As already described, many acute problems present with chest pain as a feature. This section will concentrate on chest pain that is a result of the patient suffering an acute coronary syndrome (ACS): unstable angina, non-ST segment elevation myocardial infarction (NSTEMI) and ST segment elevation myocardial infarction (STEMI). Treatment should follow the Resuscitation Council (UK) guidelines [9.12]. The pain is indicative of myocardial ischaemia or infarction, caused by a sudden and critical reduced flow of blood to the myocardium. This is due to either contraction of the smooth muscle within the wall of a coronary artery or formation of thrombus, in association with an atherosclerotic plaque that partially or completely occludes a coronary artery. The symptoms and signs consistent with acute myocardial ischaemia or infarction include:

- central chest pain, often described as dull or constricting;
- the pain often radiates to the neck, jaw, the left or both arms, or epigastrium;
- nausea and vomiting;
- pallor;
- sweating;
- tachycardia;
- dyspnoea;
- heart failure.

Although the pain described above is typical, it is not necessarily ubiquitous. The elderly, diabetics and postoperative patients may have no chest pain.

Unstable angina

The diagnosis depends on finding one or more of:

- angina on exertion, provoked by progressively less activity;
- angina occurring without provocation;

- prolonged angina suggesting myocardial infarction, but no ECG or laboratory evidence of myocardial infarction.

The 12-lead ECG may:

- be normal;
- show ST segment depression (acute myocardial ischaemia);
- show T-wave inversion (non-specific).

There is no elevation of serum cardiac troponins or cardiac enzymes.

Non-ST segment elevation myocardial infarction (NSTEMI)

The diagnosis depends on finding:

- chest pain as described earlier, usually lasting for more than 20 minutes;
- non-specific ECG changes: ST segment depression or T-wave inversion on the 12-lead ECG;
- raised plasma concentrations of cardiac troponins.

ST segment elevation myocardial infarction (STEMI) (Figure 9.7)

The diagnosis depends on finding:

- chest pain as described earlier, usually lasting for more than 20 minutes;

- ST segment elevation or new left bundle branch block (LBBB) on a 12-lead ECG;
- raised plasma concentrations of cardiac troponins.

The release of cardiac-specific troponins is evidence of myocardial infarction, but it is important not to delay treatment of a STEMI by waiting for confirmation of elevated troponin levels. Troponin levels are an important indicator of risk; the greater the value, the greater the risk of a further event or death.

Troponin levels can also be raised in many of the other acute conditions described so far including pulmonary embolism, heart failure, renal failure and sepsis.

Start treatment

All patients suffering an ACS should be treated immediately and be given:

- aspirin, 300 mg orally, crushed or chewed;
- nitrates, usually sublingual glyceryl trinitrate (GTN), unless hypotensive;
- oxygen if hypoxic ($SpO_2 < 94\%$ on air):
  - high flow initially, titrated to an SpO_2 94–98% once it can be monitored;
  - if COPD, aim for SpO_2 88–92%;
- analgesia if required, usually IV morphine, titrated to relieve pain.

Patients who have sustained a STEMI will require urgent referral for coronary reperfusion therapy, either by primary percutaneous coronary intervention

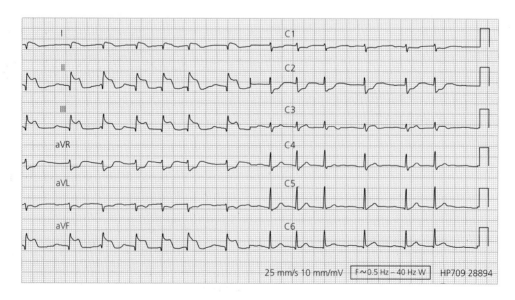

Figure 9.7 Twelve-lead ECG showing a STEMI; inferior myocardial infarction with ST segment elevation in leads II, III and aVF.

(PPCI) or fibrinolytic therapy. PPCI is the preferred option, provided it can be achieved within an appropriate time-frame. Ideally, the time from the call for help to attempted reopening of the occluded artery should be <120 minutes. For maximal efficacy, patients given PPCI will also need appropriate antithrombotic therapy. In addition to aspirin, an antiplatelet drug is given, either clopidogrel, prasugrel or ticagrelor.

Fibrinolytic therapy reduces mortality but is less effective than PPCI. However, it has the advantages of not requiring a cardiac catheter laboratory and can be delivered prehospital, which has obvious benefits if the transfer time to hospital is prolonged.

 KEY POINTS

Patients suffering from unstable angina or NSTEMI will need urgent treatment to prevent the spread of coronary thrombus:

- low molecular weight heparin or fondaparinux, subcutaneously, in a therapeutic dose;
- aspirin;
- if early PPCI is planned, consider a glycoprotein IIb/IIIa inhibitor.

If not contraindicated, a beta-blocker should be given to reduce myocardial oxygen demand and if there is evidence of heart failure, early introduction of an ACE inhibitor and a statin.

All patients should be cared for in an area with continuous ECG monitoring and immediate availability of a defibrillator. Patients should be referred urgently for consideration of coronary angiography to determine the need for coronary revascularization

Cardiac arrhythmias

Any arrhythmia can cause acute cardiovascular compromise as the effectiveness of the heart as a pump is reduced, therefore reducing cardiac output. Arrhythmias can arise for a number of reasons, the most common precipitants being:

- structural heart disease – for example, cardiomyopathy, left ventricular hypertrophy, valve disease;
- myocardial ischaemia;
- electrolyte abnormality, particularly potassium and magnesium;
- hypovolaemia;
- sepsis;
- side-effects of other drugs.

Often it is a combination of factors, for example electrolyte disturbance in the presence of longstanding left-ventricular hypertrophy.

Following the initial assessment of the patient, assuming the presence of a cardiac output, the next steps are as follows.

- Monitor SpO_2 and give oxygen if hypoxic.
- Make sure full resuscitation equipment is immediately to hand.
- Establish adequate IV access and take bloods.
- Establish continuous ECG monitoring and record a 12-lead ECG.
- Identify and treat any reversible causes (e.g. electrolyte abnormalities).

Arrhythmias can cause a variable amount of compromise depending on the exact nature of the rhythm, the heart rate and the presence of any pre-existing cardiac disease. The urgency of the situation, and hence the appropriate management, will be dictated by whether or not any adverse features are present, as these usually indicate an unstable patient who is at risk of deterioration and needs urgent treatment and senior help.

Adverse features include the following.

- Shock: systolic BP <90 mmHg, poor peripheral perfusion.
- Syncope: signifying impaired cerebral perfusion.
- Heart failure: the presence of pulmonary oedema.
- Myocardial ischaemia: chest pain or ECG changes suggesting ischaemia.

More specific management directed at restoring a normal heart rate and/or rhythm can be started once the underlying rhythm abnormality and the urgency are known. The following are based on the Resuscitation Council (UK) 2015 guidelines (see Further information).

Tachycardia

This is defined as a resting heart rate of > 100 beats/minute.

These can be divided based on the duration of the QRS complex on the ECG into:

- narrow complex tachycardias (QRS < 0.12 s) – supra-ventricular in origin;
- broad complex tachycardias (QRS > 0.12 s) – these can be ventricular in origin or supra-ventricular tachycardia with an abnormal conduction pathway.

If in doubt as to the exact cause of a broad complex tachycardia treat it as ventricular tachycardia.

Irrespective of the rhythm, any patients **with any adverse features** will need synchronized cardioversion under sedation or general anaesthesia and an anaesthetist should be called for this. Up to three shocks of increasing energy may be delivered. The starting energy level needed for cardioversion depends upon the type of arrhythmia:

- Broad complex or atrial fibrillation – 120–150 J and increase in increments.
- Regular narrow complex and atrial flutter – 70– 120 J.
- For atrial fibrillation or flutter, use the anteroposterior defibrillator pad position if possible.

If the arrhythmia is not terminated after three shocks, give 300 mg amiodarone IV over 10–20 min followed by another single shock.

If the patient **does not have any adverse features** there are other treatment options:

- Narrow complex, regular – likely to be a supraventricular tachycardia (SVT), try vagal manoeuvres (carotid sinus massage, Valsalva manoeuvre). If these fail give up to three rapid IV adenosine boluses (6 mg, 12 mg, 12 mg). If sinus rhythm is not restored, more expert help will be needed.
- Narrow complex, irregular – likely to be atrial fibrillation; give a beta-blocker IV.
- Broad complex, regular – probable ventricular tachycardia (VT), give amiodarone 300 mg IV over 20–60 min, followed by 900 mg over 24 h (via a central line).
- Broad complex, irregular – obtain expert help as it will probably be difficult to determine the underlying rhythm.

Bradycardia

This is defined as a resting heart rate of <60 beats/minute.

If there are any **adverse features** present:

- give atropine 500 µg IV immediately;
- this can be repeated until a satisfactory heart rate and blood pressure are achieved, or up to a maximum dose of 3 mg;
- if there is an inadequate response to atropine, then an adrenaline infusion or transcutaneous pacing can be started;
- patients requiring an adrenaline infusion or transcutaneous pacing will subsequently require transvenous pacing and specialist cardiology help should be obtained urgently.

If there are **no adverse features** present:

- assess the risk of deterioration to asystole. A high risk is associated with:
  - recent asystole;
  - Mobitz type 2 atrioventricular (AV) block;
  - complete heart block with broad QRS complex;
  - ventricular pause >3 seconds;
- if a high risk is present, treat as above and obtain expert help;
- if there are no high-risk features, the patient can be monitored.

Transcutaneous pacing

This can be established rapidly, but it usually causes the patient considerable discomfort and analgesia and/or sedation is often required.

- Position the pads in the conventional right and left chest positions.
- Select the desired pacing rate, usually between 60 and 90 beats/minute for adults.
- Choose the lowest energy setting if available.
- Turn on the pacemaker and gradually increase the output, watching both the patient and the ECG trace.
- A pacing spike will appear on the ECG and, as the current is increased, eventually a QRS complex. This indicates 'electrical capture'.
- Check that each QRS complex is followed by a T-wave to eliminate pacing current producing a QRS artefact.
- Once electrical capture has occurred, check that each QRS complex is followed by a palpable pulse. This is 'mechanical capture'.
- If mechanical capture does not occur, this equates to PEA. Consider other likely causes (see later).

Cardiac arrest

Unfortunately, significant numbers of patients in hospital will have a cardiac arrest either as a result of primary cardiac disease or as the endpoint of unrecognized physiological deterioration. All healthcare professionals need to be competent to deal with a patient who has had a cardiac arrest, either as a first responder or as a member of the cardiac arrest team. The details below are based on the guidelines produced by the Resuscitation Council (UK) [9.12].

Members of the team responding to a cardiac arrest call should ideally meet at the beginning of their period of duty and carry out a number of tasks, including:

- introductions by name;
- identification of skills and experience;

- allocate team leader responsibility;
- allocate roles, for example airway management, defibrillation;
- identify any deficiencies and how they can be managed – for example, if nobody is able to perform tracheal intubation;
- ensure that everyone is aware of the need for personal safety – for example, use of gloves and need for ANTT techniques;
- the need to ensure that audit is performed;
- arrangements for debriefing.

Actions on attending a cardiac arrest

On most occasions in hospital, resuscitation will have been started by other healthcare professionals before the team arrives. A standardized approach to management of cardiac arrest is used, dependent on the initial rhythm, either shockable (ventricular fibrillation/pulseless ventricular tachycardia (VF/pVT)) or non-shockable (PEA or asystole). This is summarized in Figure 9.8.

- Confirm cardiac arrest, check for breathing and a central pulse simultaneously (Figure 9.9).
- Ensure good-quality CPR (compression-ventilation ratio 30:2) (Figure 9.10).
  - Chest compressions: heel of hands in middle of lower half of sternum, depth 5–6 cm, rate 100–120/minute, ensure complete release between compressions. Use a CPR feedback or prompt device if available.
  - Ventilation: use a bag-mask alone or with a supraglottic airway device. If the skills are available, perform tracheal intubation. Ventilate at 10 breaths/minute.
  - Attach self-adhesive defibrillator pads while chest compressions are ongoing (Figure 9.11).
- Once the airway is secure, attempt uninterrupted compressions and ventilations.
- If available, attach waveform capnography.
- Plan actions for team members to minimize hands-off time if defibrillation is required.
- Stop CPR and check rhythm on monitor, the immediately resume CPR. Take less than 5 seconds.

If VF or pVT

1 Designated person selects correct energy on the defibrillator and charges defibrillator. Choose an energy setting of at least 150 J for the first shock and the same or higher for subsequent shocks.

2 During charging, continue chest compressions, warn all team members to stand clear, **except the person doing chest compressions,** and remove any device delivering oxygen.

3 Once the defibrillator is charged, warn person doing chest compressions to stand clear. **When clear, deliver shock** and immediately restart chest compressions. The pause in compressions should be less than 5 seconds.

4 There is no indication to check the rhythm or feel for a pulse.

5 Continue CPR for 2 minutes, team leader prepares for actions during next pause.
  - After 2 min, check the monitor:
    - if a rhythm compatible with a cardiac output is seen, check for signs of a circulation, such as pulse or increase in ETCO$_2$;
    - if VF persists, repeat steps 1–5.
  - After 2 minutes, check the monitor:
    - if a rhythm compatible with a cardiac output is seen, check for signs of a circulation;
    - if VF persists, repeat steps 1–4;
    - give 1 mg adrenaline IV and 300 mg amiodarone IV while performing CPR.
- Repeat the 2 minute sequence of 'CPR–rhythm check–defibrillation' while VF persists.
- Give further doses of 1 mg adrenaline every alternate shock, approximately every 3–5 minutes.
- In shock-refractory VF, identify and treat any reversible causes that may be contributing, such as hyperkalaemia.
- If the patient has a return of spontaneous circulation (ROSC), organize post-resuscitation care. This will require transfer of the patient to a critical care area.
- If the rhythm changes to asystole or electrical activity without a perfusing rhythm, switch to the non-shockable side of the algorithm (see later).

Witnessed or monitored VF/pVT arrests

This may occur when the patient is on the coronary care unit, in a critical care area or in the catheter laboratory. In these circumstances, a defibrillator is usually immediately available.

- Confirm cardiac arrest and summon help.
- If the rhythm is VF/pVT, give up to three shocks in quick succession ('stacked shocks').
- Check for a rhythm change or other signs of ROSC after each shock. If the third shock is unsuccessful, start chest compressions and follow the ALS algorithm.

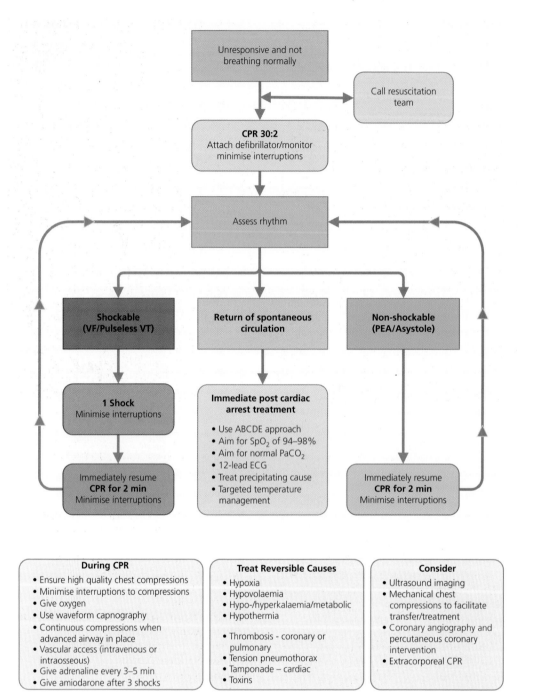

Figure 9.8 Adult Advanced Life Support (ALS) algorithm. Source: courtesy of the Resuscitation Council (UK).

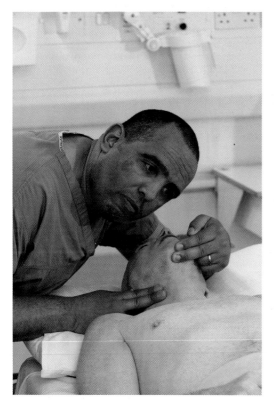
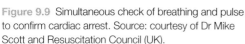

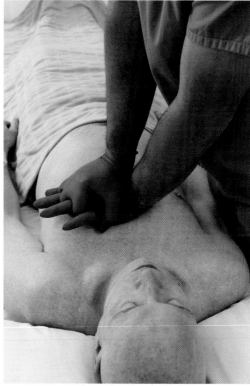

Figure 9.9 Simultaneous check of breathing and pulse to confirm cardiac arrest. Source: courtesy of Dr Mike Scott and Resuscitation Council (UK).

Figure 9.10 Chest compressions during CPR. Note hand position in the middle of the lower half of the sternum. Source: courtesy of Dr Mike Scott and Resuscitation Council (UK).

In these circumstances, the three shocks are considered the same as the first shock in the standard ALS algorithm. Adrenaline should be given, if required, after two further attempts at defibrillation.

If PEA or asystole

- Ensure chest compressions are ongoing.
- Give adrenaline 1 mg IV.
- During 2-minute CPR, secure the airway if not already done.
- After 2 minutes, check rhythm; if organized electrical activity is seen, check for signs of a circulation:
  - if there is ROSC, organize post-resuscitation care;
  - if there is no ROSC, continue CPR for 2 minutes, give further doses of adrenaline every 3–5 minutes;
  - recheck the rhythm check every 2 minutes;

  - if there is a change to VF/pVT at the rhythm check, change to the shockable side of the algorithm.
- While CPR is ongoing, identify and treat any reversible causes (4Hs and 4Ts):
  - hypoxia;
  - hypovolaemia;
  - hypo-/hyperkalaemia/metabolic disturbances;
  - hypothermia;
  - thrombosis – coronary or pulmonary;
  - tension pneumothorax;
  - tamponade – cardiac;
  - toxins – for example, drug overdose.

If resuscitation is unsuccessful, the team leader should initiate a discussion on stopping the attempt with all team members. This will require judgement based upon the patient's premorbid status, current rhythm, response so far to the resuscitation, and likelihood of ROSC if continuing the attempt.

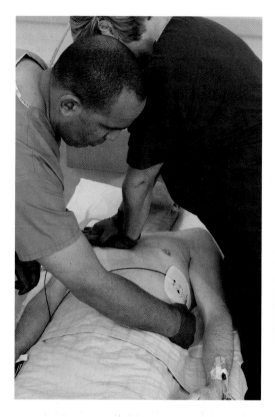

Figure 9.11 Self-adhesive pads being applied with on-going chest compressions. Source: courtesy of Dr Mike Scott and Resuscitation Council (UK).

 KEY POINTS

- Ensure good-quality CPR is performed at all times. Change the person performing CPR regularly (every 2 minutes) to prevent fatigue.
- Minimize delays between stopping compressions and delivering the shock – ideally less than 5 seconds.
- Resume chest compressions immediately after shock delivery. Even if a perfusing rhythm has been restored, a pulse may not be palpable.
- If an organized rhythm is seen during the 2-minute period of CPR, do not stop chest compressions unless the patient shows signs of life.
- In shock-refractory VF, check the position and contact of the pads.
- If there is doubt whether the rhythm is fine VF or asystole, do not attempt defibrillation – continue CPR. This may improve the amplitude of VF and increase the chance of successful defibrillation.

they are doing; if no response, give 0.5 mg atropine and further doses as required.
- Give adrenaline incrementally in doses of 50–100 µg IV rather than a 1 mg bolus. If repeat doses are required, consider an infusion.

Decisions about cardiopulmonary resuscitation

In UK hospitals, only around 20% of patients recover after receiving CPR. CPR is most likely to be effective in those whose cardiorespiratory arrest has a treatable cause, usually a shockable rhythm (VF or pVT). For patients with advanced and irreversible life-limiting conditions, for example widespread cancer or advanced heart failure, futile attempts at CPR will deprive the individual of a dignified death, or might prolong but not stop the dying process, thereby subjecting them (and those who care about them) to further suffering. In these patients, CPR should not be attempted.

All hospitalized patients who are at risk of cardiac arrest or dying should have a decision made and recorded as soon as possible about whether or not they will receive CPR. The responsibility for this ultimately rests with the senior clinician in charge of their care at the time of the decision. Case law has established that the patient **must** be involved in the

Confirmation of death occurs approximately 5 minutes after stopping CPR by confirming that there is no evidence of a central pulse and no heart sounds on auscultation.

At the end of every cardiac arrest, it is the team leader's responsibility to ensure that appropriate audit data is collected and recorded.

Intraoperative cardiac arrest

Patients will normally be monitored so there should be little delay in recognition. Follow the ALS algorithm, but consider specific changes.

- Chest compressions are effective in the prone position – do not waste time turning the patient supine.
- Try a precordial thump if a defibrillator is not immediately available.
- Extreme bradycardia or sudden asystole is most likely due to surgical stimulation causing excessive vagal activity. Ask the surgeon to stop whatever

decision-making process, unless they lack capacity for this or the discussion would cause physical or psychological harm. This does **not** mean that CPR should be offered to people in whom it would be of no benefit or that patients have a right to demand treatment that is not clinically indicated. It does mean that, where CPR would offer no benefit, the decision and the reasons for a Do Not Attempt CPR (DNACPR) should be explained to each patient in a sensitive manner.

It is also good practice to discuss a decision about CPR with all the healthcare professionals caring for the patient and, with consent, the patient's family or other carers. If the patient lacks capacity, the decision must be discussed with the family, carers or other representatives as soon as is practicable and appropriate. When a decision about CPR is made, it must be recorded in the patient's health record (and usually also on a dedicated form), along with the reasons for reaching this decision, and be communicated to all those involved in the patient's care.

A DNACPR decision applies **only** to CPR for cardiorespiratory arrest. All other care a patient requires must be provided and be of the highest standard; this may include oxygen, antibiotics, nutrition, hydration, analgesia and sedation. A DNACPR decision must not lead to the withholding of any other care or treatment [9.13]. Finally, decisions about CPR should be reviewed regularly to allow a change of decision, in either direction, in response to changes in a patient's clinical condition.

Ideally, all patients approaching the end of their life should be involved in a positive process of advance planning that allows them, with guidance from healthcare professionals, to agree goals for their care and choose what interventions they would or would not wish to receive in the event of deterioration. Considering treatment options in this way is more acceptable to patients and healthcare professionals than focusing on one treatment (CPR) when it is not on offer. Such an approach is currently being adopted in developing a process and decision document for use in the UK.

Reduced conscious level

This may be due to a number of causes. The treatment priorities are to:

- establish and maintain a patent airway;
- ensure adequate oxygenation and ventilation;
- support or restore an adequate circulation;
- assess the GCS score.

Then proceed to determine the cause of the depressed consciousness. Some of the more common causes, and their management, are outlined below.

Hypoglycaemia

This is most likely in patients with diabetes receiving oral hypoglycaemic agents or insulin treatment. It can occur in the perioperative period if there is inadequate carbohydrate intake or absorption but normal doses of medication are continued, and in those developing sepsis. Patients with poorly controlled diabetes may become symptomatic at what would otherwise be considered normal blood glucose concentrations. Other groups of patients at risk are those with hepatic failure, who have impaired hepatic gluconeogenesis during starvation, and those who have had a gastrectomy. The brain is dependent on a constant supply of glucose for energy and so untreated hypoglycaemia has the potential to cause irreversible brain damage.

The presenting features depend on blood sugar concentration and are due to autonomic stimulation and inadequate glucose delivery to the brain:

- autonomic – sweating, tachycardia, tremor, hunger: patients taking beta-blockers may not have any of the autonomic signs or symptoms of hypoglycaemia;
- inadequate cerebral glucose delivery – delirium, reduced GCS, seizures.

Details within the patient's medical history may raise suspicion of the diagnosis, and a conscious patient may describe the classic symptoms listed above. The diagnosis is confirmed by checking a capillary blood glucose concentration. All patients with a decreased GCS should have a capillary blood glucose checked as part of their initial assessment.

Start treatment

The key aims are to increase the blood glucose concentration back to normal levels, and prevent further hypoglycaemic episodes.

If the patient has a patent airway, is breathing and conscious:

- give oral glucose gel, for example Glucogel© – glucose is rapidly absorbed across the buccal membranes;
- obtain IV access;
- the oral glucose alone may not be enough, and a bolus of 250–500 mL 10% dextrose IV may be needed.

If the patient is unconscious

- Ensure a patent airway and adequate ventilation.
- Obtain IV access and give 25–50 g of dextrose as an IV dextrose solution:
  - 50% dextrose is often stored on resuscitation trolleys, but causes phlebitis;
  - 10% dextrose is preferable as this causes less irritation.
- A rapid recovery is often seen.

Calculating the dose of dextrose in grams from percentage:

$$concentration(\%) \times 10 \times volume(L) = dose(g)$$

e.g. 500 mL of 10% solution

$$10\% \times 10 \times 0.5L = 50g$$

Investigations

- Twelve-lead ECG to check for any myocardial ischaemia or arrhythmia.
- Blood tests, including FBC, U&Es, blood sugar and blood cultures.

Once the blood glucose concentration has been restored to normal, the symptoms should have resolved. If there is ongoing neurological impairment, an alternative explanation should be sought. Further episodes can be prevented by:

- the patient taking an oral diet:
  - immediate and slow-release carbohydrate, for example sugary drink and toast;
  - consider altering dose of regular diabetes medication;
- the patient not taking oral diet or not absorbing enteral nutrition:
  - intravenous insulin and dextrose infusions either as a sliding scale or an 'Alberti regime' according to local guidelines;
  - stop normal diabetes medication until normal oral diet has been resumed;
- all patients must have frequent monitoring of capillary blood glucose until the 'at risk' period is over.

Opioid narcosis

Opioids form a key part of the management of moderate and severe acute postoperative pain. A variety of different opioids is in common use and they can be administered via a number of different routes – for example, oral, IV, intrathecal or epidural. There is also a wide interindividual variability in the metabolism and elimination of opioids, which leads to the

potential for overdose. The elderly, patients with obstructive sleep apnoea and those with altered renal function are particularly at risk.

Specific features of opioid overdose include the following.

- *History:* receiving opioids, elderly, abnormal renal function.
- *Hypoventilation:* particularly reduced respiratory rate.
- *Pupils:* 'pin-point' in appearance.

Start treatment

- Ensure an adequate airway, breathing and circulation.
- Establish IV access if not already in place.
- Give naloxone, in 100–200 µg boluses IV, until an adequate conscious level and respiratory rate are restored.

Naloxone also reverses the analgesic effects of the opioids. The aim is that with careful titration, the harmful side-effects can be reversed without antagonizing all the analgesia.

The effects of naloxone are relatively short-lived (approximately 20 minutes). Therefore, if long-acting opioids have been given, such as morphine, or opioids have been given intrathecally, repeat naloxone doses or an infusion may be needed, as well as adequate monitoring, which may necessitate admission to a critical care unit.

Stroke/intracranial haemorrhage

A stroke may occur for a number of different reasons including, but not limited to:

- atrial fibrillation – emboli from atrial thrombus;
- severe hypotension – due to haemorrhage or sepsis;
- a period of hypoxaemia – due to respiratory depression from opioids;
- intracranial haemorrhage – due to anticoagulation with heparin;
- related to surgery – emboli following carotid endarterectomy.

The clinical features and appropriate management depend upon the extent and the location of the cerebral damage:

- if there is infarction of a large volume of cerebral tissue, or a large intracranial haematoma, the patient's GCS will be reduced and the patient may not be able to maintain a patent airway;
- small areas of infarct may give rise to only localized motor or sensory deficits with a preserved GCS.

Start treatment

- Ensure an adequate airway, breathing and circulation.
- Give supplemental oxygen; if $SpO_2 < 94\%$, aim for 94–98%.

Priorities

Following the initial assessment and stabilization, the priorities are as follows.

- An urgent CT scan of the head to confirm the diagnosis (Figure 9.12). This may necessitate intubation and ventilation to be performed safely:
  - some centres are performing thrombolysis for ischaemic strokes confirmed by CT scan within 3 hours of onset of symptoms – in these cases time is of the essence;
  - thrombolysis may be contraindicated in the postoperative period.
- If intracranial haemorrhage is excluded by CT scan, 300 mg aspirin should be given as soon as possible.
- Control blood glucose concentrations. Use a glucose and insulin infusion if needed; a target of 4–11 mmol/L is recommended.
- Blood pressure control is only indicated if there are other problems, such as intracerebral haemorrhage or myocardial infarction, or if thrombolysis is planned.

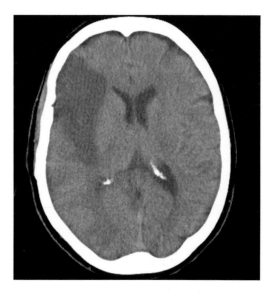

Figure 9.12 CT brain showing large low-density area in the right frontoparietal region, consistent with an ischaemic stroke.

- Conscious patients should have a swallowing assessment; nasogastric feeding should be started within 24 hours in patients unable to swallow safely.
- Involve the acute stroke team early.

If the CT scan shows an intracranial haemorrhage, the patient will need to be discussed with the local neurosurgical unit to determine if surgical management will be beneficial. If the patient is on anticoagulant therapy, there may be some difficult decisions about the relative risks and benefits of continuing or stopping treatment. Further management will depend on the neurosurgical opinion.

Status epilepticus

Status epilepticus is defined as seizures lasting more than 30 minutes, or frequent seizures over 30 minutes without a return to consciousness. The aim of treatment is to terminate seizures as quickly as possible because of the high mortality associated with them, and this usually requires intravenous antiepileptic drugs or, if refractory, general anaesthesia. Early expert help is therefore essential.

The common causes of status epilepticus include:

- unstable, poorly controlled epilepsy;
- *acute brain injury*: stroke, tumour, subarachnoid haemorrhage, trauma, hypoxia;
- *previous brain injury*: trauma, neurosurgery, arteriovenous malformations;
- *CNS infection*: encephalitis, meningitis, abscess;
- *metabolic abnormalities*: hypoglycaemia, hyponatraemia, hypocalcaemia, uraemia;
- subtherapeutic antiepileptic drug levels in known epileptics;
- *withdrawal syndromes*: alcohol, barbiturates or benzodiazepines;
- eclampsia of pregnancy;
- febrile convulsions may precipitate status epilepticus in young children (three months to three years of age).

Start treatment

- Clear and maintain an airway. This may be difficult. A nasopharyngeal airway is often very useful due to clenching of the jaw during the fit.
- Give high-flow oxygen via a facemask with reservoir.
- Establish IV access and take blood for immediate glucose analysis.
- Correct hypotension with IV fluids.

- Start antiepileptic therapy IV:
  - first-line therapy, IV lorazepam up to 4.0 mg;
  - if IV access is not possible, diazepam 10 mg PR (this may already have been given by paramedics prehospital).

If seizures continue

- IV phenytoin 15 mg/kg at a rate of ≤50 mg/minute.
- ECG monitoring is essential as there is a risk of bradycardia and heart block.
- IV sodium valproate 10 mg/kg at a rate of ≤100 mg/minute (followed by 1.6 g over 24 hours).

Refractory status epilepticus

- Induce and maintain general anaesthesia with tracheal intubation. This will require expert help.

Investigations

- Plasma glucose, U&Es, calcium, magnesium, FBC, therapeutic drug levels, toxicology screen, arterial blood gases.
- Septic screen, including lumbar puncture if CNS infection suspected.
- CT scan: the possibility of intracranial pathology is high if this is the first presentation of epilepsy.
- EEG.

As soon as seizures are controlled, refer the patient to a neurologist.

Reduced level of consciousness secondary to hypoxaemia or hypovolaemia

The brain requires a constant supply of oxygen for its normal function. Both hypoxaemia and hypovolaemia will compromise cerebral oxygen delivery. Both of these abnormalities should have been detected and treated during the initial ABCDE assessment of the patient, and some signs of increasing cerebral function may be seen within minutes of appropriate management.

It must be remembered that hypoxaemia or hypovolaemia may themselves be due to another problem; for example, hypoxaemia may be due to pneumonia or pneumothorax, and hypovolaemia may be the result of intra-abdominal bleeding postoperatively. Initial measures may temporarily restore cerebral oxygenation, but definitive treatment needs to be targeted towards the underlying problem, for example intubation and mechanical ventilation, while the pneumonia resolves with antimicrobial therapy, drainage of the pneumothorax or return to theatre to stop the bleeding.

FURTHER INFORMATION

British Thoracic Society Standards of Care Committee Pulmonary Embolism Guideline Development Group. British Thoracic Society guidelines for management of suspected acute pulmonary embolism. *Thorax* 2003; **58**; 470–484.

Lim W, Baudoin S, George R, *et al.* British Thoracic Society guideline for the management of community acquired pneumonia in adults: update 2009. *Thorax* 2009; **64** (supplement III); iii1–iii55.

National Institute for Health and Clinical Excellence. *Clinical Guideline 68. Diagnosis and Initial Management of Acute Stroke and Transient Ischaemic Attack (TIA).* London: NICE, 2008.

National Institute for Health and Clinical Excellence. *Clinical Guideline 94. Unstable Angina and NSTEMI: The Early Management of Unstable Angina and Non-ST-Segment-Elevation Myocardial Infarction.* London: NICE, 2010.

O'Driscoll B, Howard L, Davison A. British Thoracic Society guideline for emergency oxygen use in adult patients. *Thorax* 2008; **63** (supplement VI): vi1–vi68 (to be updated in 2016).

Ramrakha P, Moore K, Sam A (eds). *Oxford Handbook of Acute Medicine*, 3rd edn. Oxford: Oxford University Press, 2010.

Resuscitation Council (UK). *Adult Advanced Life Support Manual*, 7th edn. London: Resuscitation Council (UK), 2015.

[9.1] http://bestbets.org/
This web site contains best evidence topic reviews for emergency medicine. Many of these are relevant to anaesthesia and critically ill patients.

[9.2] www.nice.org.uk/CG50
Recognition of and response to acute illness in adults in hospital. July 2007. The National Institute for Health and Care Excellence (NICE) guidelines – you must read this if you are interested in this topic. Soon to be updated.

[9.3] www.rcplondon.ac.uk/projects/outputs/national-early-warning-score-news
Documents from the Royal College of Physicians on the application and interpretation of NEWS.

[9.4] www.institute.nhs.uk/safer_care/safer_care/situation_background_assessment_recommendation.html
Detailed information including videos of the use of SBAR.

[9.5] www.tracheostomy.org.uk
Organization aiming to reduce preventable deaths from mismanagement of blocked tracheostomies and laryngectomies.

[9.6] www.brit-thoracic.org.uk/document-library/clinical-information/asthma/btssign-asthma-guideline-2014
The British Thoracic Society and the Scottish Intercollegiate Guideline Network guidelines on management of asthma.

[9.7] www.survivingsepsis.org
Comprehensive web site run by the European Society of Intensive Care Medicine aimed at improving recognition and management of sepsis.

[9.8] www.resus.org.uk/anaphylaxis/emergency-treatment-of-anaphylactic-reactions/
Resuscitation Council (UK). Emergency Treatment of Anaphylactic Reactions. Guidelines for Healthcare Providers. Amended 2012.

[9.9] www.nice.org.uk/guidance/cg134/resources
NICE guidance on assessment and referral after emergency treatment for anaphylaxis.

[9.10] www.nice.org.uk/guidance/cg169
Guidelines from NICE on acute kidney injury: prevention, detection and management.

[9.11] www.renal.org/Clinical/GuidelinesSection/AcuteKidneyInjury.aspx
The Renal Association web site with the current guidelines for management of acute kidney injury. 2011.

[9.12] www.resus.org.uk The Resuscitation Council (UK).
This site contains the current UK guidelines for management of acute coronary syndromes, cardiac arrhythmias and cardiopulmonary resuscitation.

[9.13] www.resus.org.uk/dnacpr/decisions-relating-to-cpr/
Joint document from the Resuscitation Council (UK), Royal College of Nursing and British Medical Association covering all aspects of decision making relating to CPR.

Index

Page numbers in *italics* refer to illustrations; those in **bold** refer to tables

Clinical Anaesthesia: Lecture Notes, Fifth Edition. Matthew Gwinnutt
and Carl Gwinnutt.
© 2017 John Wiley & Sons, Ltd. Published 2017 by John Wiley & Sons, Ltd.
Companion website: www.lecturenoteseries.com/anaesthesia